Notes from a Child Psychologist

Notes from a Child Psychologist

Louis Propp, PsyD

ROWMAN & LITTLEFIELD
Lanham • Boulder • New York • London

Published by Rowman & Littlefield
An imprint of The Rowman & Littlefield Publishing Group, Inc.
4501 Forbes Boulevard, Suite 200, Lanham, Maryland 20706
www.rowman.com
86-90 Paul Street, London EC2A 4NE

British Library Cataloguing in Publication Information available

Library of Congress Cataloging-in-Publication Data

Names: Propp, Louis, 1949- author.
Title: Notes from a child psychologist / Louis Propp, PsyD.
Description: Lanham : Rowman & Littlefield, [2024] | Includes index.
Identifiers: LCCN 2023047878 (print) | LCCN 2023047879 (ebook) | ISBN
   9781538190371 (cloth) | ISBN 9781538190388 (paperback) | ISBN
   9781538190395 (epub)
Subjects: LCSH: Child psychopathology—Case studies. | Family psychotherapy—
   Case studies.
Classification: LCC RJ499 .P7167 2024 (print) | LCC RJ499 (ebook) | DDC
   618.92/89—dc23/eng/20231229
LC record available at https://lccn.loc.gov/2023047878
LC ebook record available at https://lccn.loc.gov/2023047879

I would like to dedicate this book to my family: Kristin, Jascha, Abigail, Jedediah, Augustus, Hannah, Jules, and Riis. A special dedication to my wife, Kristin, for all her help and support.

Contents

Preface: A Lifetime of Play

I worked as a child psychologist in Vermont for more than thirty-six years. The community where I lived and practiced was mostly white and blue collar, with roughly 15 percent of children under eighteen below the poverty level. It was primarily rural.

During that time, I saw children as young as three years old and often continued to see them as they matured into adolescents and adults. In some instances, I saw my patients with their own babies or young children years after they'd been my patients. I even worked with different members of families by doing therapy with brothers, sisters, and relatives of patients.

As a therapist in a small community, I became a pivotal part of the lives of my patients and their families through my sessions. In my relationships with them, I saw how destructive family patterns often repeated and negatively impacted the children and adolescents under my care. I witnessed how, with treatment, it was possible to harness the power of a child's or adolescent's family to help my young patients form their own identity and not have to repeat these patterns. I decided to write this book to tell the stories of how children and adolescents can discover themselves through therapy and how parents and caregivers can help them in this discovery.

Each story in this book features fictionalized, composite characters I've created based on real patients I saw in that small Vermont community, and each revolves around a different psychological problem that I treated. In these stories, children, adolescents, and other family members attending their sessions talk about their lives—their challenges and desires—while I tease out my patients' conflicts and problems. The reader sits with me in my office and learns about my patients and their families by listening to the play interactions and therapeutic dialogues and hearing my thoughts as a therapist. In this way, I hope that my experience as a child psychologist becomes your experience and that, along the way, you begin to understand what it must be like for a child or adolescent to be in a room with a therapist.

The stories show how my therapy involves a delicate balance of understanding my patients' behaviors and family patterns. Each story focuses on a particular patient's challenges and situation. Each person's story is different. In these stories, the treatment I describe is the one that best fits that particular patient. The therapy I do is about the art of appreciating and understanding the psychological themes of my patients and their families. I work with this knowledge to help my child and adolescent patients make changes.

The medium of play is central to the therapeutic conversation I have with children. It is the joy and driving force of the therapy I do with them. The rhythm of play is what creates a fun relationship with younger patients and makes them want to return to therapy. I use play to assess, evaluate, and treat my patients. Through the meditative quality of play, I am able to help my child patients regulate and balance their behavior struggles. I reframe a child's aggression and competitiveness into empathic and cooperative interactions through their play. The creative aspect of play helps me better understand the underlying actions of my younger patients.

As a child psychologist, I have to understand and keep up with my patients' play and toy culture. Sometimes I need to learn about a toy character through my patients, and we research the figure together to better understand its characteristics. I've read up on video games to learn about their content and themes. In certain cases, I've explained the content of the game to parents and caregivers to help them understand its appropriateness for their child. As a child ages, their play evolves into complex games with more rules. They also begin to play with ideas and positive and negative thoughts about their parents, families, and caregivers.

As teenagers, my patients begin to develop their own stories. I encourage them to question the influence of their family patterns on their problematic actions. In their stories, my adolescent patients begin to think: What have I learned from my parents? What do I like—and what don't I like—about my parents' choices? They start to realize in their therapy that they have choices, too. In my relationships with teenagers, I help them decide what behaviors they want to change. In later childhood, trust is established when adolescents feel comfortable sharing, processing, and playing around with their ideas and thoughts about family. I have found in my treatment that older children find more meaning in what they say to me as opposed to what I say to them. In my therapeutic relationships, I create an atmosphere that encourages teenagers to explore their families' psychological dilemmas.

The treatment stories in this book show the powerful influences families and caregivers have on young people. With children, I work at developing a trusting relationship with a parent or caregiver so I can better understand the family story. Through therapy, I help my child and adolescent patients uncover their personal theme and how it does or doesn't fit into the family story. I engage parents and caregivers so they can help their child's own story evolve. The support of a parent or caregiver in therapy allows a child to reflect on, understand, and validate their actions.

I hope these stories will help illuminate the underlying struggles of children and adolescents and the fact that their behaviors have meaning. Their playfulness has vibrancy. Moreover, being sensitive to them, understanding them, and listening to them helps them feel good about who they are. Adults sometimes want to forget about their younger life because of their own conflicts, disappointments, and guilt and have trouble participating in their children having fun. I hope this book helps readers accept their own childhood experiences and find that there is joy in playing and having fun with children.

I have been fortunate to work in a state where all children have insurance that covers mental health services. This allowed me to see a diverse group of children and families. I believe the range of psychological problems of the children and adolescents I have treated have universal themes. I believe readers will see in these stories the art of my therapeutic relationship, and the underlying depth of family interactions. I hope some of you will feel inspired to pursue a career working with children and families. I hope these stories will help parents feel comfortable bringing their children in to see a child therapist.

Special Confidentiality Statement

As a licensed child psychologist, I am bound by ethical and legal concerns. I am not able to disclose the identities of the children, adolescents, and families I have worked with in therapy throughout my thirty-six-year career. I have to respect my patients' confidentiality. In this book, I wanted to show the kinds of psychological problems I have seen in my practice. To do this, I have used the genre of creative nonfiction to construct fictional actors. These made-up characters are conglomerates of the many patients I have seen in the past. I have created stories to demonstrate ten different cases and problems. The struggles and conflicts are real. However, all characters and their stories are totally invented. I have not revealed any actual patient I have seen. I attest to this confidentiality statement to assure that the security of the patients I have seen in therapy is completely protected.

Acknowledgments

I want to thank my family, my friends, and others who offered suggestions and recommendations and encouraged me to keep writing.

I extend my gratitude to the following people: Morgan Arlcth, Isabelle Bleecker, Eric Braun, Scott Burg, Catherine Dubios, Geri Fuhrmann, Mark Kerr, Christine Lin, Denise Main, Ben Presskreischer, Helene Presskreischer, Peter Pierre, Carlie Scribner, Michelle Weyers, and Lori Yunger.

Thanks to my favorite authors:

Toni Morrison who, in her writings, reminded me that the search for ourselves is always there for us to discover.

Fyodor Dostoevsky for his use of dialogue and the presentation of multiple narrative voices to explain psychological dilemmas.

Oliver Sacks for a framework to guide the structure of this book.

Chapter 1

Does Ricky Have Depression?

PRESENTING PROBLEMS

Ricky was an eleven-year old boy when he began treatment with me. I evaluated him and he shared his frustrations about school. He said he had trouble paying attention in class. Autumn, his mother, was confused. She was getting conflicting messages about Ricky's behavior. The school believed he was acting out. His primary care physician said he might be depressed. Rick, his father, didn't see his son as having any problems. He was upset. He blamed everyone else.

Autumn was Ricky's best advocate and was the one who brought him in for his sessions. She agreed with me that attention deficit disorder (ADD) was an appropriate diagnosis for him. Autumn understood that, in addition to his therapy, Ricky needed a medication intervention to improve his attention. Rick had trouble believing that his son needed to be on a pill, even though he might have had the same problems Ricky had when he was his age.

Ricky over time felt he benefited from our treatment and medication. The cognitive behavioral interventions I taught Ricky helped him focus. He successfully used the strategies in his classes. Ricky in time learned to work with the medication and was able to pass his academic classes. As high school ended for Ricky, his parents became an integral part of his treatment. They accepted his personal struggles and understood his difficulties with attention.

TREATMENT STORY

Autumn called to set up an appointment for her eleven-year-old son, Ricky, who had recently been suspended from school. A difficult meeting at the school had left her and her husband concerned about their son. I scheduled

1

a visit for her and her husband, Rick. Sometimes, I like to have both parents come in first without the child in order to gather a clearer understanding of the child's problem.

Autumn and Rick arrived on time, and Rick, a rather large man with red hair and red beard, strode into my office and sat on the couch. The back of his shirt read, "Rick's Construction," with a stylized logo. Autumn followed him in, handed me the clipboard with the completed intake information, and sat next to him. Slightly shorter than Rick, she was a dark-haired woman, wearing nurse's scrubs with a name stamp from our local hospital. I reviewed the forms, signed the consent to treatment, and started the session.

Autumn began by telling me that Ricky's pediatrician, Dr. Thomas, had referred them to me. He had prescribed antidepressant medication for Ricky. "But Rick and I don't know if we agree. Ricky is happy and energetic at home. He is constantly on the move."

Rick, who had been sitting rigidly on the couch, interrupted. "Something's going on with that school," he said. "The teacher is always on the kid's back. I think she's a problem."

Autumn shot him a look and continued: "We decided to come here. We had a terrible meeting with his school."

"You mentioned that on the phone," I said. "Tell me about the meeting." I wanted to understand how she and her husband perceived this school interaction. I could see they might have differing opinions. I was hoping to establish some agreement about Ricky's behavior and the reasons for his recent suspension.

"It was uncomfortable," she said. "He has only been in school for a couple of months, but it felt like they already saw Ricky as a real problem! His teacher said he refused to do his work."

"Is that why he was suspended?" I asked.

"No," Autumn said. "He left the classroom without permission. When he didn't return, they launched a school-wide emergency search. He was found hiding in a janitorial closet crying. The principal said he had to suspend him. He made an unsafe choice. They recommended we get him help."

I asked for background information about other school years. Is this the first time he left the classroom? What frustrated him enough to make such a decision?

She said, "All his past teachers would offer Ricky extra help if he didn't get his classwork done, or they would send it home. We made sure he completed it. Ricky told us he didn't like this teacher. She makes him stay in the class and finish his work. He told us it makes him late for recess."

I realized Dr. Thomas must have observed Ricky's frustration, sadness, and negativity and wanted to help, so he prescribed medication. I was not sure if Ricky was depressed, but I knew Dr. Thomas would be receptive to input from me. We had worked together often in our small community. I mentioned this to Autumn and Rick.

"Ricky told Dr. Thomas he hated school," Autumn said.

Rick blurted out, "The doctor's a quack! They always give kids pills!"

"Medication can sometimes be an important part of treatment, but there may be other ways to help Ricky," I assured Rick. I was concerned that Rick was taking his son's behavior personally. Rick and Autumn appeared to each have their own perspective on his behavior.

I continued the intake by asking whether depression was a pattern in the family.

Neither parent said they had been on antidepressant medication, nor did they report a family history of depression. His mother insisted, "I don't see depression. He seems content at home. He helps with the household chores. Sure, I have to remind him what to do. I have to make sure he finishes. He and his six-year-old brother Jordan mostly get along. I think something else must be going on. I believe it has to do with school. But I will give him the medication if you and the doctor think it's best."

His father barked, "He doesn't need a drug; he just needs to do his schoolwork."

I decided to try and engage Rick more. I could see he cared about his son but was having trouble understanding his son's problem. I asked him about his work and his experience in school.

He perked up. He said, "I run my own business! I have enough work to keep me busy year-round. I do remember having problems in school. I hated sitting still. I was put into a building trades program in high school. I liked it and didn't have to be in a classroom all day."

I asked him what he thought about Ricky's behavior in school.

"I told Ricky that, if he does better in school, I'll take him hunting," he said. "My father had me out in the woods as soon as I could walk."

Autumn smiled as she nudged him. "You were probably older than two, but I agree it would be a good idea for you to take Ricky in the woods. But not until he completes the Hunter Safety course. You enjoy hunting, and it would give you and Ricky some quality time together."

When I asked about her schooling, Autumn said she was a good student and completed a two-year nursing program.

I wanted to learn more about Ricky's behavior. What was he like at home? His father had struggles in school, he couldn't sit still, and he impulsively made statements during our conversation. I began to think Ricky may not be depressed. I wondered if he was more like his father and had trouble with paying attention in school?

His mother said, "Ricky plays video games. He can play for hours. When he can't sleep, I have caught him playing his games." When I asked if she knew the content of the games, she said, "They're just games. He picks them out."

Next, I asked about Ricky's after-school routine.

"He is usually outside with the neighbor's son after school," Autumn said. "The boy's mother watches both my boys until I get home from work. When I get home, Jordan plays in his room while I help Ricky with his schoolwork."

"How does that go?" I asked. "How does he do with his homework?" I wanted to understand how he handled learning and his level of frustration when she worked with him.

"It has been a challenge!" she admitted. "He sits at the kitchen table while I make dinner. He starts with how he hates school. How his teacher makes him miss recess if he doesn't do his math paper. Then he complains about having to do his homework. I tell him he has to stay put until he gets it done. Finally he settles down and does it. What should be ten minutes of homework takes three to four times that long with all his fussing." I could see the frustration on her face as she recalled this routine—her mouth tightened and she shook her head slightly. "Here's what I don't understand," she added. "After all my prodding to get the work done, and after the ordeal he goes through, his teacher insisted at the meeting that he hadn't handed in most of his homework. I know he's doing it because I sit there with him until it's done!"

I felt I had gathered enough of an understanding of the family patterns, and I ended the session. I believed Ricky might have some attention or learning issues. His attempts at doing his schoolwork frustrated and upset him, which made him feel sad. Dr. Thomas certainly picked up this feeling. I set up a time for Ricky to come in. His mother agreed to bring him, as his father said he couldn't manage the time due to his work commitments. I thanked them both for sharing their family backgrounds.

* * *

I easily identified Ricky in the waiting room with his bright red hair like his father's and Lego T-shirt. A wiry figure, he sat at the children's play table noisily putting large block pieces together. I smiled at him and his mother and directed him into my office. As soon as he entered, he immediately noticed the Lego constructions on the second-to-top shelf and quickly walked toward them, pointing.

He shouted out, "Who made those?"

"You can look, but don't touch," I said before he could grab one. I explained that the Lego buildings had been put together by other children. "If you had made one, you wouldn't want other children to touch or mess up what you made."

He was genuinely interested in the projects. But now, instead of grabbing one, he eyed them carefully. He asked again who made them.

I talked to him about child therapy. I said that part of coming here was playing with the toys and games and drawing. I pointed to the children's drawings on the board in front of where he was standing, which was above the children's play table. He turned from looking at the Legos on his right to see what I was showing him. I told him the Lego projects and drawings were made by other children who also come here for therapy. I explained that they come here to play and talk about their problems at home and in school. I told him I couldn't say who made what because I had to protect their privacy. If he decided to make something, I wouldn't be able to tell anyone else except his parents that he made it.

My patients had been working on a hover vehicle theme. I told Ricky that the rule was that the projects had to be made with no wheels.

"Would you like to make one?" I asked.

"I do want to make one," he said.

To help him organize his space, I pulled out the chair under the children's play table and placed the box of Legos next to his seat. Right away he started raking his hand through the Legos. I handed him a flat, long piece and suggested to him that it could be a good base to start his hovercraft. As he worked, I told him I would place his project on the shelf like the others so he could finish it at a later session.

He appeared to be engaged and enthusiastic about participating. I had to stay vigilant. He picked up the box of Legos and was about to dump them on the table when I grabbed it. I said, "Please be careful and just take handfuls."

I remained attentive and observed his play. I wanted to watch how he attended to a high-interest activity. How did he work on a fun project? What were his planning and organizational skills? Could he stay focused?

He fumbled through the box of Legos, gathering a bunch of the blocks in one fist. I suggested that he put them next to the flat piece I gave him. His search for parts seemed to be random, without any criteria for size, color, or purpose. He laid another handful of blocks on the table and started building. I soon realized his building was random, too—he was simply clicking blocks together. I redirected him back to the hovercraft. I suggested he add some small pieces to the baseplate piece. His play activity was scattered and disorganized. He was having trouble even completing a fun project. I pointed this out to him. No wonder he was having difficulty learning and attending in school. I asked him, "Do you have trouble finishing your schoolwork?"

He nodded: "Yes!"

I intermixed our conversations about school and home while helping him gradually finish his project. I did this because he pouted when I brought up school. But he enjoyed manipulating the small blocks. Putting together his version of a hovercraft seemed to soothe him. I had to offer him instructions and advice for his building. He accepted the suggestions and didn't protest.

I wondered what he did at home. Did he play with his brother? What did he do for fun? I said, "Your mother told me you liked video games."

"I play outside with Jordan," he said. "He's not good at video games, but he likes watching me play. I like the fighting and shooting games."

I asked if his parents knew about the games.

He said, "No! I pick them out."

I glanced at the clock. I wanted to have time to include his mother in the session. I said, "Let's get your mother." As soon as he heard this, he ran out to the waiting room and returned with her.

His mother placed herself on the couch. She sat in a rigid position and had a worried look on her face as she watched him. He had jumped back on his seat at the play table and began pawing loudly through the box of Legos. I challenged him to work on his vehicle.

While he worked, I described to his mother my observations about Ricky's distracted and chaotic play behavior and told her what he said about his difficulties paying attention in school. "I believe his problem with focusing frustrates him," I said. "I think he might have left the class because he couldn't tolerate being so upset."

"I think I know what you mean," Autumn said. "I have to tell him many times to finish things. He needs constant reminders. Getting him ready for school in the morning is quite the task."

I told her that I would like to evaluate Ricky's behavior further with a standardized assessment tool. It had both parent and teacher versions. I would score the forms and interpret the findings based on norms for his age. I showed her the parent questionnaire, and as she looked it over she said, "I would score him high on this. He doesn't pay attention."

She and I observed Ricky haphazardly building with the Lego blocks while listening to our conversation. I asked how he was doing with his construction.

He said, "Good."

I said that I agreed with her—he was easily distracted. I believed his classwork was probably difficult for him to concentrate on. I wouldn't be surprised if his acting out at school was related to his difficulties paying attention.

"Do you think he has ADD?" his mother chimed in. "I was wondering about this. I read an article about attention problems in children, and the descriptions reminded me of Ricky."

"That is the purpose of the assessment," I said. If both parents and his teacher score him high for attention problems, it would validate my observations. She consented to using the evaluation.

Before the session ended, I suggested to his mother that she check the content of the video games he plays. I talked to her about limiting the amount of his screen time. This may help him sleep better, I said. I gave her a list of violent video games and age-appropriate games. Ricky listened intently to this parenting discussion.

* * *

The completed assessment forms were in our mail slot early enough that I could score them for our next meeting. I found Ricky met criteria for attention problems both from his mother and teacher. He had a combination type of ADD that includes concentration challenges and impulsivity. I believed his difficulty with attending to low-priority (for him) school tasks frustrated him, which could lead to him impulsively acting out. He did, however, have the skills to be attentive when he played his high-interest video games. The teacher didn't note any learning concerns, and he wasn't in the clinical range for depression.

I could hear Ricky banging the blocks in the waiting room before his next visit. I knew he was excited to come in and work on his hovercraft When I invited him into the office, I attempted to slow the process down. I talked to him about his partly finished project as I placed it on the table. I put the box of Legos next to where he seated himself and sat next to him.

I wanted to help him structure the task of completing his project. "What if you divide the craft into a front, middle, and back area?" I suggested. "Maybe you could use different colors for each section."

He said, "I want to use white for here, then red, and blue here." He moved his finger along the areas from front to back as he indicated the colors.

I suggested he take the different colored pieces he wants to use and put them in piles according to color. He followed along, showing no problem listening and responding to instructions while creating his construction. He assembled the small, colored bricks on the hovercraft without focusing on any particular area. He seemed to relish connecting the Legos together. *A sense of accomplishment*, I thought. I gently coached him and acknowledged his success.

He turned his head and pointed to another craft on the shelf. "Maybe I should make one like that," he said.

He was clearly distractible, but I encouraged him to finish what he was doing. "Yours will look just as good," I said. "I can't wait to see what it looks like when you finish. Maybe you should work on one area at a time."

"I like that!" he said and started placing the small white bricks on the front.

With the structure of the play established, we developed a rhythm of working on the project and talking about how this past week went. I wanted to establish the importance of having fun playing together while also having him reflect on his behavior. I asked, "How did school go this week?"

"Not bad!" he said.

"Did you complete your classwork?" I asked.

"I think I did," he said. "I'm almost done. Can I show my mother what I made?"

I suggested some spots where he could add bricks and told him that after he finished he could get his mother. I wanted to see if he could finish one task before he started another. He followed my direction and finished off the red section of his hovercraft. We admired it together, and I could see that he was quite proud of it. With that, I asked him to go into the waiting room and get his mother.

They returned, and Autumn sat back on the couch. Ricky sat at the table and dumped a bunch of Legos on top of it. He was about to begin another building adventure. I proposed he organize the pieces in piles according to their color like he did before, and I gave him another baseplate to use. I suggested that he build another construction while his mother and I talked, and he quickly became engaged in a new project. I noticed, though, that he listened to our discussion.

As at our last visit, Autumn wore nurse's scrubs but this time in purple. She crossed her legs but leaned forward on the couch, eager to learn what I had ascertained about her son. I started by explaining that Ricky didn't meet the criteria for depression. The assessments indicated, however, that Ricky had problems with attention, and my observations working with him confirmed that. His attention challenges led to his problems in school.

"But wait," Autumn said. She looked at Ricky working on his Lego project. "I have a question. If he can't pay attention, how can he play his video games for hours?"

"He has a high interest in playing his video games," I said. "The classroom is different—doing classwork is not a top priority for him. He can pay attention to things he likes and may even show impressive focus on those things. This is typical for children with attention problems."

She commented, "What about the medication he's on? It was prescribed for depression. Should we get him off that?"

I explained that the release she signed during the intake allowed me to talk with Dr. Thomas about Ricky. I would tell him about my findings. Several months ago we were at the same conference in Burlington on using medication and behavior strategies for attention problems, and we even talked about the importance of working together on these cases. I told her I would contact Dr. Thomas before Ricky's med check the following week in order to discuss his medication. I was hoping he would start Ricky on a more specific medication to target his attention problem. Then I would like to observe him on it so I could see its effectiveness.

I told Autumn that, in conjunction with a change in medication, I would like to develop a treatment plan for Ricky's attention issues. I looked over at him and said, "When you come here, I can help you with focusing and homework strategies."

He said, "What do you mean?"

I pointed to his hovercraft. "Look at what a great construction you made!" I said. "Just like you made this vehicle by breaking it into sections and using different colors for the sections, you can use that strategy for your home-work." I explained to Autumn how she could break up his homework into smaller tasks and maybe use a red folder as trigger for his homework to be handed in the next day.

* * *

Dr. Thomas and I had a productive consultation. He agreed with my assess-ment and prescribed an extended release stimulant that would last through the school day and about an hour afterward, so Ricky could complete his homework. He would gradually discontinue the depression medication. We agreed to keep each other informed.

When the time came for Ricky's next appointment, I didn't hear him in the waiting room like I had before. When I went to get him, he was quietly look-ing at the Lego magazine. He would have been on the medication for about two weeks by then.

As he came into my office, he noticed the new Lego displays on the shelf and commented, "Those are good! They are Minecraft figures, right? That one is a Creeper. I know that one is Pig. That one looks like an Enderman." He pointed to each creation as he named it, but he didn't reach out to grab or touch them. "I want to make one!"

I was curious to observe if there was a difference in the quality of his play since being on the medication. Could he focus better? Would he be more amenable to planning strategies?

He insisted he wanted to put together his favorite Minecraft character, a Ghast. I was worried because I had seen the figure before. I knew it would be complicated to construct with Legos. The character consisted of a large, square head/body structure held up with six thin legs. I was worried he wouldn't be able to hold up the figure with the legs. I tried to persuade him to build another figure, but he persisted: "I want to make it."

I wasn't going to change his mind, so I relented and went with it. Watching him undertake this complex project would give me an opportunity to assess his planning and attention skills. Hopefully he wouldn't become too frus-trated. I proposed that he break up the project into tasks, as he had with the hovercraft.

He immediately became engaged. "I'm going to pick out small pieces for the legs and make six piles. The body I will make with larger pieces and put them in another pile."

I helped him gather the blocks into the different piles. I expressed my concern about how he would be able to attach the legs to the large body section.

"I think I have an idea," he said.

I watched as he began building the body and head section. As he had finished most of this part, I gave him a gentle challenge: "I still don't see how you are going to attach the legs."

"Watch," he said.

I did. I began to notice that he was leaving an indentation on the base of the head and body section. I asked if this was where he was going to connect the legs.

He smiled. "Yes!"

He completed the six legs and connected them to the head/body base. I observed that he maintained his attention. He followed basic instructions and organized his work. He also developed a plan in response to my presenting him with a query about how he would connect the legs to the large body section. I believed he had the skill set to learn focusing strategies with the addition of the medication helping to improve his attention to task.

I asked him if he thought the medicine was helpful. He said, "Yeah! It helps." I said I never thought he would be able to put together a Ghast. I commended him for staying focused and doing such a great job. I said I would like to place it on the display shelf.

He was pleased with how well the figure turned out. He maneuvered the item so it could stand on its own. "I did it! I made it."

I strategically placed it on the shelf and asked him how school was going. Did he notice any difference in his classroom attentiveness?

"I look at the teacher," he said. "I do my work. I take a break. I don't let the other kids bother me. It's better."

"Let's have your mother come in," I said.

He calmly stood up and came with me to escort his mother into my office. He pointed (without touching) to the construction he had just completed. He explained a little about the figure to his mother.

Autumn was impressed. "That is quite a good Lego figure. I like what you did!"

I said to her that he had an exceptional ability to build Lego projects compared to other children his age. Again, he listened intently as I told her that I noticed he stayed on task while he built the figure. I said he told me he feels he is doing better in class. I asked what she thought.

"He doesn't complain about school," she said, smiling. This was surely a relief for her. "His teacher met me at the office today when I picked Ricky up for his appointment. She said he is better in class and is getting his schoolwork done."

"That's great," I said. "What about at home?"

"I can see the difference at home," she said. "He seems to get his home-work done quicker. I used your idea about colors to organize things and gave him a red folder for his homework. I break up his homework into tasks. When he finishes, he gets a reward of screen time."

I said it appears that Ricky had been making good progress. Next I brought up the topic of video games. I expressed my concerns about the content of the games he had been playing. I asked if she'd had a chance to look at the lists of games I gave to her.

His mother said that she had made some parent decisions after reviewing the list and talking it over with his father. "We decided to put away some of the games until he is older. We have set new rules. He has a regular bedtime with a story, he can only play age-appropriate games, and his screen time is limited. On school nights, he only gets screen time after he finishes his homework."

I turned to Ricky, who was still concentrating on his Lego creation. I knew he was listening to the conversation, so I asked, "What do you think about the new rules, Ricky?"

He turned around and faced us and said, "It doesn't bother me. I like the rules."

* * *

Throughout the school year, Ricky continued to show improvement. He consistently turned in his homework with the trigger of the red folder. He built many fun creations while learning focusing strategies, staying on task, completing one item before starting another, breaking up his project, organiz-ing his work space, and learning to develop a plan. While playing, he and I would also talk about how he could use these strategies in school. His father, although not as physically involved, seemed to agree with the treatment plans, at least according to his mother.

Over time, his mother developed a positive rapport with Ricky's teacher and said to me, "His teacher sends me e-mails. Ricky stays up to date on his classwork. She said he is not a problem in class. She said he has become a better student."

Toward the end of the school year, his mother began to worry about the challenges he may have during the summer. Should he continue taking the medication? He would have less structure. What about next year, when sixth grade has different teachers for each class?

I proposed that she think about a plan for the summer. We could talk more about Ricky's transition into sixth grade when he gets his class schedule. This usually happens a couple of weeks before school starts. I advised her that it would be important for Ricky to have a fun vacation and not worry about school. I provided her with a list of local weekly summer camp programs.

In order to evaluate his progress, I scheduled a couple of sessions for him over the summer. She set up a med check with Dr. Thomas before school ended. We set up a parent session for the end of his summer vacation.

Ricky's summer sessions were both upbeat. He played with the Legos but was more intent about telling me about his camp experiences. He didn't want to talk about school. His mother told me, "He really enjoyed camp. He would come home excited with many stories to tell. Dr. Thomas said we could try not giving him his medication on the weekends. He wanted us to see how he would do without it when he had less structure. It definitely helped during the week and for camp. His father studied with him so he earned his Hunter Safety certificate. His father wants to take him for the youth hunting weekend in the fall."

I said I would see Ricky again when school started. I asked her if Rick would still be able to come to our parent session in two weeks. She said he was planning on it.

When that parent session came, I could tell something had changed. Rick burst into my office with Autumn following. I hadn't seen him in a while. I wanted to be friendly and hoped to talk about Ricky's success, but it was clear something was bothering him.

He said, "Look, Doc! I never had to take a pill when I was his age. I made it through school. Now I have a job that pays well."

I calmly explained to him Ricky's difficulties with paying attention. I reminded him how distracted and frustrated Ricky was with school. I attempted to convey how the medication had helped.

His father grumbled, "Will he have to be on a drug for the rest of his life?"

Autumn seemed to be aware of his underlying concern. "Why don't you tell him about your helper and high school friend?" she asked. "You have done a lot for him."

Rick said, "A guy I know, Jim, said he had ADD in high school. He was given pills. He told me that's why he became an addict. He got help. I gave him a job. He's been with me for many years now. Now he doesn't drink, do drugs, or anything. He's a good father. He said he would never give his kid a pill!"

I finally realized where Rick was coming from. I tried to reassure him by explaining that Ricky's medication was being prescribed, and he was under careful observation by Dr. Thomas and myself, not to mention Rick and Autumn. In addition, he is learning focusing strategies. Eventually the goal would be to reduce or eliminate the medication as his attention improved.

His father begrudgingly accepted what I was saying. "I get that the pill has helped my son. It sounds like it's not a life sentence. I see we got to work to get him off the drug."

Autumn asked if I had suggestions for other interventions. "One of my coworkers told me about her son being on a 504 plan. She said he had ADD. What is a 504?" she asked.

I explained the basics of the Section 504 disability law to his parents. A plan could be developed for Ricky to support his learning. Accommodations could include less distracting seating in the classroom, homework monitoring, motor breaks, and weekly teacher feedback. A 504 plan is a coordinated effort between the parents and teachers to improve a child's educational experience based on the child's disabling condition.

Autumn expressed her interest in exploring such a plan during the upcoming school year, but Rick was frustrated again. I noticed his face begin to redden. "What the hell!" he bellowed. "Now you're saying my son is disabled."

Autumn and I attempted to reassure him that this plan would be in place to help his son. We reminded him that Ricky's attention problems affected his school performance. But Rick was uncomfortable with the conversation.

"Are we done yet?" he asked. He was tuning out.

As the session was nearing the allowed time anyway, I summarized the content. I scheduled another appointment for Ricky with his mother. Rick shifted about on the couch as I spoke, and then he got up and abruptly left my office. I said I would see Autumn after a couple of weeks when school had started. She seemed satisfied. But I was left with the feeling that Rick was still not happy with his son being in treatment.

* * *

My suspicions were confirmed when the next appointment was canceled, and the one after that. In fact, I didn't hear anything from the family for a couple of months—well into the school year. Autumn called to tell me that Ricky asked to have one last session. I became concerned. What had happened? I hoped all was going well and he didn't need further help, but I suspected something else was going on. I scheduled a session for the following week.

As I neared Ricky in the waiting room, he appeared subdued. This was unusual because I could always tell when he was in the waiting room. At previous appointments, he would be noisily constructing items on the children's play table abutting my office. His productive activity carried through to my office even though it was slightly muted by sound machines and music. I missed that playful presence. I could tell something was different.

Autumn looked up from reading a magazine.

Ricky slowly turned toward me. "Is it my turn?" he asked.

He accompanied me into my office and looked at the display shelf. He asked, "What are the kids building?"

I said to him the project was to put together a small Lego building and include a figure inside it. He seemed reluctant to participate. I knew this was his last appointment. Could I get him to talk about what was going on?

He sat at the children's play table and grabbed a handful of Legos.

I asked him if he could tell me what he has been doing since we last met. He haphazardly put random pieces of the Legos together, but he seemed unsure how to proceed. I could tell he wanted to say something and was struggling to get it out.

I gave him time, and he gradually shared his circumstances. He said, "My father said if I get good grades he will take me hunting."

"And how are you doing with your grades?" I asked.

"My grades are good."

"So does that mean you will be going hunting?" I knew the youth hunting weekend was coming up soon.

He perked up a little. "Yeah! Dad and I have been target practicing. He gave me a rifle. He's been showing me how to track a deer."

I asked if the medication was still helpful.

He said, "Dad said I don't need to take the pills. He said hunting would help. He said I don't have to come here."

When Autumn came in, she confirmed that she believed Ricky benefited from therapy. I could tell she wanted to leave open the possibility of future interventions. But she needed to respect his father's authority in the family. I was pleased to know that Ricky's father was becoming more involved.

She said, "Since Ricky has been practicing shooting with his father, he has been doing okay in school. I still feel the medicine and counseling helped. His father never liked the idea of his son taking a drug. He father wanted to handle the problem in his own way. I see the difference in their relationship. They have bonded on hunting."

At the end of our time, I said, "I wish you good luck and hope you get your first deer with your dad." I informed his mother that she could contact me at a later time if treatment was needed.

* * *

About a year and a half later, Autumn called after the school's long winter vacation. She sounded concerned. "The holidays have not been good," she said. "Ricky was sad and didn't seem himself. He mostly stayed in his room. He is failing all his subjects."

I asked her what had happened since we last met.

She said, "Ricky made it through seventh grade, but he had to go to summer school in order to pass. He said he missed having fun over the summer. We thought that maybe spending the summer going to school might motivate him to put more effort in eighth grade. But it didn't work. He said he wanted to talk with you again."

I scheduled a session for the following week.

Ricky had grown taller and heftier since I had last seen him. He walked confidently into my office and sat straight up in the chair. He looked at me and got right to the point: "I want to go back on the pills. I did much better in school when I was on them. I told my mother they helped."

I was impressed by his candidness. I knew his mother would be comfortable with this decision. What about his father?

"I think he would agree," Ricky said. "We got to talk a lot when we hunted together. He was different when we were outside in the woods. He even asked me if the pills really helped. I told him the truth: they did. And I told him about the things I learned by coming in here."

"What did he say about you coming here today?" I asked.

"My father thought it would be a good idea. He told me he wished he could have gotten some help when he had trouble in school."

This was a good sign. Though Rick had seemed stubborn at first, he obviously cared about his son and was willing to listen. And he was willing to change his mind.

Ricky looked over the recent constructions displayed on the shelf and said, "I missed coming in here. I liked building and talking about things." He shared his frustrations with school and how he has to stay after to catch up with his classwork.

I explained that we would have to develop a new therapy plan. "You seem better able to talk about your problems now," I said. "You may not be as interested in Legos, but we could always play a game while we talk." Ricky nodded and smiled.

When we invited Autumn into the office, she was quite clear about her goals. She said, "I want him to do better in school. He said the medication helped him pay attention. His father admitted Ricky did his best when he was on the medication and in therapy."

I asked if Rick was more understanding of his son's difficulties with paying attention. Is he still as worried about the medication?"

"After their hunting incident, Rick saw Ricky's attention problem for himself," she said.

"Hunting incident?" I asked. As before, Ricky listened intently to our discussion.

Autumn explained, "They went out hunting. They had been in the woods for a while and were both tired. All of a sudden, Ricky dangerously fired his gun without thinking or looking for something to shoot at. His father is a stickler for gun safety. He said he lost it and yelled at him. Ricky started crying and said he couldn't help it. He thought he saw something and just wanted to fire the gun."

She informed me that, after this, she and Rick had many discussions about Ricky, the medication, and school. She said, "I think we are both in complete agreement now. Rick understands the reason for the medication. He even understands that the medication is part of a therapy program to help Ricky with school. Rick had similar problems in school, and he said he probably wouldn't have graduated if it weren't for the hands-on building program he was in."

We talked about goals. Autumn would contact Dr. Thomas to restart the medication. I would submit a 504 request to the special educator. I would specifically recommend a tutoring program to help him catch up with his classwork. I would note that his attention disorder affected his ability to complete his work, and that treatment had resumed.

Ricky was eager to reengage in therapy. Instead of Legos, we played chess and checkers. He was quite good at checkers and enjoyed our matches. He talked about the techniques he used to complete his schoolwork and how he managed to stay attentive. His mother and even his father participated in some of the sessions. His father made a positive comment about how he believed the medication was helpful. At the end of the school year, his mother shared that he had passed all his classes except for English, which he would retake over the summer.

Ricky continued to participate in therapy on a less-regular basis during high school. He continued on the medication, but only for school days. In his junior year, he was placed in a hands-on program in design and manufacturing. We had our last session around that time. Ricky was taking a short-acting and lower dose of the medication. He was much better able to complete his homework and didn't require other supports. Since he was in a more hands-on program for about half the school day, he and his mother felt he didn't need the 504 plan anymore. The 504 high school coordinator agreed. I said I could always submit another plan if necessary.

Several years later, I was at Home Depot on a weekend when I heard someone calling my name. "Dr. Propp! Dr. Propp!" When I turned around, I saw a rather large, red-haired young man with a wispy red beard. Due to my position in the community, I am always careful about acknowledging others unless they say something to me first. I do this to protect patient confidentiality.

"Hi, it's me, Ricky," he said.

An image came to me about a Lego Ghast creation, and I realized who I was talking to. I felt a smile spread across my face. "Ricky!" I said. Since we were in close proximity to each other, I asked him how he was doing.

"I'm getting some materials for Dad. I graduated high school. Look at this." He turned around so I could see the back of his shirt, which read "Rick's Construction."

He showed me a list he'd made on a sheet of notepaper, which was well organized by different pieces of wood broken down according to their dimensions. Ricky had grown up and had learned some successful skills. We shook hands and said, "Nice to see you," knowing we had shared something very special in the relationship we had had in the past.

CHALLENGES AND REFLECTIONS

Ricky's mother Autumn accepted my findings that Ricky was not depressed as his physician had stated. I shared with her how disorganized his play was. I explained that he was distracted even when he would play fun activities. I found him to be enthusiastic and not unhappy. Autumn concurred with me. Rick, his father, had his own strong opinions. It was a challenge to enlist him in the treatment. He had trouble with the idea of adding medication to help Ricky improve his attention. This presented a difficult balancing act among the parents, Ricky, and myself. I had to keep the focus of my treatment on what would benefit Ricky.

The other challenge I had in this case was to establish a diagnosis that fit with Ricky's behavior. I did this by observing and watching his actions during our sessions. I validated what I had seen with a standard assessment scale. The quality of Ricky's play showed the trouble he had with attention issues; he was easily distracted and was unable to organize and even put together a fun play construction. His behaviors were classified under the category of an attention deficit disorder. Autumn was on board with this diagnosis. She was comfortable trying a medication intervention. Rick was reluctant but went along with his son being on a pill.

Ricky became invested in our treatment and learned different focusing skills. He discovered that the medication along with the techniques he learned in therapy were helping him. His mother supported our treatment. She worked with the school to set up a special plan to help him catch up with his class assignments. Rick became increasingly annoyed with his son being in treatment. He decided to take him off the pills. He didn't think he needed therapy. Rick thought he could help him by teaching him to hunt. I thought this would be the end of my treatment with Ricky.

Ricky, however, believed that the treatment and medication had been helpful. He found that without the combination of therapy and medication he became unsuccessful in school again. He couldn't concentrate on his schoolwork. After a while, Ricky requested to return to therapy. His mother brought him in. His father had his reservations.

As a teenager, Ricky took more responsibility for his treatment. He knew what worked best for him. His mother saw his maturity and his ability to change his behavior. Rick started to participate in family therapy when Ricky was in high school. He began to understand his son's problem. I think this happened because Rick admitted he went through similar attention issues when he was in school.

This sensitivity and appreciation of Ricky's concentration difficulties by both parents offered him needed support. At the end of my treatment, I believed Autumn and Rick understood my plan. They realized I was teaching Ricky specific focusing techniques to help him become less dependent on the medication.

Chapter 2

Rainbow Dash

PRESENTING PROBLEMS

James presented as a socially awkward eight-year-old second grader. He had difficulties connecting with his peers. James was the kind of child who wouldn't notice if he was being bullied. Arlene, his mother, worried about his lack of relationships at school. He resisted social interactions, she said. She reported to me that his teacher had concerns about James socially. He was behind in some academic areas, especially with reading. Arlene wanted James seen in therapy to better understand his problems.

In order to bond with him in therapy, I had to find a way to communicate with him. His behaviors led me to believe he was on the autism spectrum. I attempted to walk Arlene through the steps to have him evaluated by the school team to validate my clinical assessment. Arlene felt some relief after he was diagnosed with autism. She was worried, however, that having this disorder would impair him for life. I addressed her concerns at a later time in family treatment with her and James.

James had established a trust in our therapeutic relationship. As a teenager, he allowed me into his internal life and his social media interactions. In his secret online role, he expressed himself as a girl named Jamie. He shared with me in therapy that he wanted to transition from male to female. In family therapy, James opened up to his mother. He told her he wanted to be called Jamie and to be referred to as *she*. Jamie continued to include Arlene in her gender discovery. Ken, her father, didn't attend any of her sessions. Jamie developed a strategy in her treatment to tell her father about her interest in transitioning from male to female. She remained focused on one major transition in her life at a time, a characteristic of her autism. Jamie was motivated to complete her gender change. She engaged her parents to support the psychological and medical changes she needed to undertake.

TREATMENT STORY

Arlene, a tall, dark-haired woman, brought her eight-year-old son, James, to his first appointment with me. As I handed her the intake packet, she gave me a manila envelope. "This is a letter from Mrs. Rice, James's teacher," she said.

I looked at James. He was sitting right next to his mother in the waiting room but made no attempt to make eye contact. His head was bent over an animal magazine, his dark hair hanging over his face. He was absorbed in some pictures of penguins. I tried to engage him by asking, "Do you like penguins?" But he didn't move his head.

This appeared to frustrate his mother, who instructed him, "James, please put the magazine back and go with the doctor."

The boy dutifully listened to her. In a mechanical way, he got up and put the magazine on the rack. He still hadn't made any attempt to acknowledge me. I directed him to accompany me into my office.

When he entered the office, he didn't show any excitement about the toys and games as most children do. I was expecting he would sit at the children's play table. Instead, he remained standing and stared at the bulletin board on the wall above the table. He was looking at a series of My Little Pony pictures drawn by some of my other patients. He appeared to be mesmerized.

I tried to talk with him about the pictures. "Those pictures were made by children who like My Little Pony characters." I shared that other children come in here and like to draw. I tried to help him feel comfortable and safe. I asked, "Do you like them?"

He finally responded with a halting speech pattern. His slow and hesitant statements made him seem anxious. He said, "I have—all kinds—of Ponies—at home. I—collect—them."

I pulled out the small bench from under the play table and prompted him to sit down. All the while, he was still fixated on the pictures. In fact, I was concerned he would miss the seat because he continued to stare at them. Finally, in a slow, robotic manner, he sat down. I positioned myself to his right in an adult chair at the corner of the table so I could avoid making too much direct eye contact. I noticed he had difficulty tolerating this. I asked, "Do you know about My Little Pony?"

His lips and mouth moved while the other parts of his face were almost frozen. He stated, "Rainbow Dash—she—is—my favorite. I—like—her colors."

I was intrigued by his communication style. Not only did he hesitate between words, but he articulated with minimal intonations. He made no eye contact. I believed this was likely due to a combination of anxiety and social communications problems. I continued to engage him about his favorite toy.

"Do-you-want me-to-tell-you-about-her?" he said, slightly more smoothly. He looked up at the drawing board and briefly turned his head and glanced at me. I think we were finally making a connection, and he seemed a little less worried. "What do you like about Rainbow Dash?" I asked.

"Rainbow Dash, is a female, Pegasus pony. I, wish, I was her. She has a cutie mark, of two blue lightning bolts. All Little Ponies, have cutie marks."

His speech flowed a little more now. He was becoming more relaxed. However, he was steadfast and had to finish his sentence. Because of this, I was mindful not to interrupt him. I attempted to entice him to play with the other toys and games in my room. He had no interest. I knew that for me to learn about him, it would have to be through his specific toy interest and not through the other toys and games I usually engage children with.

"Tell me more about Rainbow Dash," I encouraged.

"Rainbow Dash is my favorite Pony. She is, really nice. I like, her the best. I had her, for a, long time. Her tail, is like a rainbow," he said.

Because James had shown an interest in the pictures my other patients had drawn, I decided to see if I could get him to express himself through drawing. I said, "I would like to learn more about your special pony. Maybe you could draw a picture of what Rainbow Dash looks like." I took out the box of colored pens and pencils and some paper and placed them in front of him on the table.

He glanced at me and said, "Someday, you could meet, her." I believed he was trying to make a social connection by wanting to share his special toy with me.

I said, "I would like to meet her."

He picked out the colored pencils he needed from the box and strategically placed them close to the sheet of paper in front of him. His long, thin fingers gracefully maneuvered the pencil as he meticulously drew light, sharp lines to designate the outline of a pony. He then went over the lines to make them darker. His rendition was quite accurate. He didn't use the eraser.

He took some time to finish the outline and said, "This is, Rainbow Dash. Now, I am going to color her in."

He started to fill in the outline with color, being careful and precise about staying within the confines of his outline. I commented, "I have learned a lot about Rainbow Dash from you." It was time for his mother to come into the session, so I said, "You could show your mother the picture you are working on." I told him I wanted to talk with his mother about how he was doing at home and at school.

Arlene placed herself on the couch in close proximity to James. She wore pants and a button-down shirt neatly tucked into her pants. She clasped her hands on her lap and sat up straight so she could see what James was doing. She admired his picture. She said, "He likes to draw. But most of the time, he plays by himself with his toy pony figures. If he isn't playing with them, he's on the tablet his father gave him. I try to get him to eat with me; sometimes he refuses to stop what he is doing. It becomes a battle, but if I say I will take away what he is playing with, he comes to the kitchen table to eat."

"I see that you parent him with clear and direct rules," I said. "I was hoping I could ask you some background questions." James was absorbed in completing his picture. I said, "After reviewing the intake form, I see that Ken visits regularly. I would like to get some more information how the two of you co-parent."

Arlene said, "I have been the manager of a local auto parts store since James was born and Ken left. I feel like I am a single parent. His father is no help."

"What sort of work does he do?" I inquired.

She said, "Ken does coding for a computer firm. He provides us with good financial support, which is definitely a help. He has no understanding of how to relate to children. When he visits, he only interacts with James when they're talking about computer stuff."

I asked, "What is the visitation arrangement?"

She said, "He visits every weekend and stays in the spare room."

Usually a child visits a parent at their household, so I was curious about their agreement. "Why does Ken stay at your household?"

"This works best," she explained. "It started when James was a baby. Ken came to my house and would just be on his computer working. He had no understanding of how to care for an infant. I mostly took care of James when he came on the weekend. During the week, I put James in childcare so I could work. I'm the manager of the NAPA Auto Parts."

"Has James been to his home?"

"Once, and that was it!" she stated. "I brought James over to his apartment, which is about an hour drive, when he was about two. Dirty dishes and empty glasses were left all over the place and within James's reach. The place was a mess. I didn't feel safe letting James walk freely. We left after he had ordered takeout food, which James barely touched. Since that time, Ken has continued to come to our house every weekend."

I observed that James was still busy drawing and seemed oblivious to our conversation.

I mentioned that Mrs. Rice had requested that James be evaluated by the special education team. She was concerned about his learning and social problems. She wanted him assessed to see if he was on the autism spectrum. I shared with Arlene that I was wondering about autism myself. I said, "In my time with him, I observed the difficulties he had relating to me, his hesitant speech, and his problems with communicating."

She said, "I was thinking about that myself. I searched the internet and found a lot of material about kids on the autism spectrum. The descriptions sounded like James: limited social relationships and fixed toy interests. He does the same thing every day, and when he speaks he doesn't look at me and stops or hesitates. Sometimes I can't follow what he is saying."

That was why I was curious about his father. I said, "It's not uncommon to find social communication problems that tend to be patterns in families."

"In a way, his father is socially odd," she said. "He has worked at the same place he has since he finished his computer programming degree. He has no friends. He comes at the same time and leaves at exactly the same time every weekend. He always eats the same thing. I can predict when he goes to bed. He never talks unless I am the one who starts the conversation. In a way, they are like two peas in a pod."

"Are you concerned about school?" I asked.

"Yes, very much so," she said. "James is struggling with school. He doesn't have any friends. He doesn't seem interested in learning anything. He never talks about school." She paused and looked at her son, who was happily working on his drawing. "Maybe I worry too much," she added.

"I can see from Mrs. Rice's letter that she has similar concerns to yours," I said. "She is worried because he doesn't talk in class, even when she calls on him. He sits by himself at lunch. His reading is below grade level. She thinks that having him tested will provide some answers."

Arlene said she would commit herself to pursuing the school evaluation. She wanted help to better understand her child. I asked if she wanted James to continue coming in for therapy. I said I could work with him on his social skills, offer her parenting suggestions, and coordinate with the school. She welcomed the idea.

I looked over at James. He had just finished coloring in his picture. I said, "What a nice picture of Rainbow Dash! Would you like me to hang it up? Or you could bring the drawing home if you want to."

"Bring it home," he said.

"Would you like to come back?" I asked.

He said, "Can I bring Rainbow Dash, too?"

He had established some social trust with me. He wanted to show me his special pony. I said, "It would be all right with me if you brought her as long as your mother agreed." She said she did.

* * *

When James came to his next session, he had his backpack with him. He brought it into my office and placed in on the couch. He unzipped the pocket and pulled out a toy pony and said, "This is, Rainbow Dash. She, is my favorite. I want, to be her. She came today."

In order to help him develop better social rhythm, I knew I had to have the play intervention become more interactive. I thought we could do this by making up stories. I set the stage for the first story by including his favorite pony in the theme. I asked, "Would you like to make a story about Rainbow Dash making friends?"

He said, "I would like that."

"Okay," I said, "I will help you with the story."

I placed the barn in the sand table and dumped the farm animals near it. He watched and held his pony figure in his hand. I coached him. "I wonder if Rainbow Dash can become friends with horses, cows, and other farm animals."

He followed my lead by holding Rainbow Dash over the barn and saying, "This is, a story, where she, becomes friends, with animals." He moved his pony over to the pile of farm animals.

James hadn't touched any of my toys yet. I asked him to help me place the farm animals around the barn. He picked up each individual farm figure with his thumb and index finger and gently placed it around the barn. While working on the scene together, his pony toy was close to him on the child's bench. When we completed setting up the farm animals, he picked her up and held her over them and said, "These are cows, pigs, and horses who live at the farm."

I became aware that as he began to trust me more his speech was less tentative. But I had to prompt him to interact within the story. I asked him, "What happens in the story? How do they become friends?"

He responded, "She stopped the rain." He held his pony character above the scene with his long fingers, and with his other hand he sprinkled sand over the barn and animal figures.

I wanted to see if he could add more content to his story. I asked, "How could she stop the rain?" Then I wondered, "How did they become friends?"

He continued to hold her up and said, "Her magic stopped the rain. The animals and Rainbow Dash became friends. She helped them. She stopped the rain. She is the best."

* * *

As our sessions continued weekly, putting together stories became an integral part of our therapy time. James enjoyed making up different stories using the figures he had in his backpack. He became familiar with the toys I introduced from my selection. The dialogues in the stories helped his social rhythm. His speech became more fluid, and he paused much less. Over time, I didn't have to remind him to use more content in his tales. He included more details and showed conflicts between different characters.

During our parent time, James would often retell his story to his mother. Arlene liked listening. She commented about his improved social abilities and noted that he was more talkative at home. He interacted with her when they would sit and eat together. This hadn't happened before.

After a few months, Arlene shared that the school testing had confirmed the autism diagnosis. She had a school meeting with James's teacher and other staff on his educational team. She said, "James was given a number of specific learning and social goals. I researched on the internet how to parent a child with autism. I joined a parent chat group."

I was curious and asked, "What did you learn from your research?"

She told me, "I would have to assist him with socialization." She had already set up regular playdates with one of his classmates. This worked because Jaylen, the classmate, was the daughter of her friend. Jaylen was quiet and shy, too. Arlene enrolled James in an after-school computer gaming program, thinking this would help increase his social interactions.

James's interactive skills improved over time. He was less socially anxious. He said he played My Little Ponies with Jaylen. He never forgot Rainbow Dash when he came to his sessions. Arlene said that Mrs. Rice told her he was participating more in class when she called on him.

* * *

I saw James regularly throughout his elementary school years. His mother was her son's strongest advocate. She was particularly concerned that in the third grade he was reading at about a grade and a half below where he should be. We talked about his interest in picture books and whether he could be taught by using a more visual approach to learning how to read. She pushed for this at school, and he was placed in a different reading program. By fifth grade she reported that he was reading graphic novels and was now close to his grade level in reading.

During James's middle school years, I didn't see him as often for therapy. He was taller with shoulder-ength hair, and his stance wasn't as rigid. Because he didn't have many friends, he didn't have the usual peer pressure drama early teenagers talk about in therapy. He came about once a month for therapy. During our sessions, he would draw different anime figures. He had become a much better student. When we talked about his social contacts, he told me he only associated with Jaylen. He didn't like anyone else. He said, "I play animal games with her on the computer. We both play our favorite female characters. I call mine Jamie."

I didn't realize why he had chosen a female character named Jamie until I started seeing him again more consistently in high school. Arlene initiated the increase in meetings after she expressed her concerns in a session with James. She said, "He mostly stays at home on the computer or reading graphic novels. I do take him with me when I go to visit with Jaylen's mother. I worry that his social limitations will affect his ability to move out of the house and live on his own. Will having autism get in the way of James holding down a job?"

James didn't appear concerned. I reassured Arlene that having autism shouldn't place limitations on his plans. He had some job strengths, he had been responsible in school, and he maintained above-average grades. His computer skills might lead to a potential career choice. We changed our therapy goals to explore his ideas about work and his preferences for the future.

James changed where he sat in my office. Instead of drawing while sitting at the children's play table, he placed himself at the left corner of the couch close to the table. We had more direct conversations. I tried to help him look at how his interest in computers could be a potential career choice for him. We discussed how if he worked on programming, he would have limited social contacts. He admitted he didn't like dealing with a lot of people.

"I don't talk with anyone at school except Jaylen," he said. "We eat lunch together." He paused, and added, "I do have friends on the internet. I chat with them every day. I have been friends with Calvin for a long time. I text and chat with him the most. He lives in England."

I was glad he felt safe enough with me to share more about his private social life. He had shared about playing online games as a female animal character with me before. At this point, however, he was talking about more in-depth relationships on social media. I wanted to understand the quality of these relationships.

He disclosed to me, "I started chatting online with Jaylen. It began while we played animal games together. We would play with others on the internet. I met Calvin then."

* * *

James had been at the high school for a couple of years and was a sophomore. I continued to see him on a monthly basis. Since he was used to our therapeutic relationship, we could easily pick up where we left off in our monthly meetings. His mother would often touch base with me toward the end of the session to fill me in on James's home and school life. He had revealed more about his online friendships in our sessions over time. I learned that this kind of social communication worked better for him. He didn't seem to feel as anxious about interacting socially on the internet.

He said, "I like having online friends. I don't have to answer right away. I can take my time to respond when we chat. I don't have to look at them if I don't want to. It puts less pressure on me. When Jaylen talks to me at lunch, I feel like I have to say something right away. This can be too much. Sometimes, I don't want to say something. When I text, I can wait and respond, and I don't have to look at them."

Since James didn't directly socialize with anyone other than with Jaylen, I wondered about his social judgment on the internet. He told me he ignored his peers at school. In the past, he seemed to be oblivious to whether or not he was being picked on.

He informed me, "I only chat with friends I have known for a while. I play games online with them, and we talk. Calvin just introduced me to a new friend. I feel okay talking with him because he is a friend of Calvin."

"What sort of information about yourself do you share with your online friends?" I asked.

James said he gives limited facts about himself. "I only tell them I live in Vermont. I give no other personal details. All my online friends know me as Jamie. They think I am a girl."

"Isn't that the name of the character you used when you played the animal games with Jaylen?"

"Yes, it is! When I started playing online animal games, I decided to name my character Jamie. It was the easiest name I could think of with the same letters as my name," he said.

He seemed excited to talk about this. I wondered about his female identification. "Why do you want your online friends to think you are female?" I asked.

He shared, "I feel happier being Jamie. I like when my online friends refer to me with the pronoun *she*."

I was intrigued and asked, "Do you let your online friends actually see you? How do they know you as Jamie?"

He said, "I comb my hair over my face. I found some of my mother's makeup and put it on my cheeks. I wear this long pretty shirt that looks like a dress. All my online friends think I'm a girl when they see me. I like it."

As we were nearing the end of the session, I asked, "How much of your internet life have you shared with your mother?" I said that sharing some of this might help her understand his social interactions better. "I have certainly learned more about your social life," I said. "Maybe it would help your mother not be as worried about you socially."

"I don't think I'm ready," he said. "Let me think about it. We can talk more about it next time."

I told him I would respect his confidentiality. I realized that he had shared some intimate social details.

* * *

In a follow-up meeting, James was ready to share his social media life with his mother. The two of them sat side by side on the couch. He nervously fingered his hair, while Arlene kept her hands in her lap and listened carefully. He did not make eye contact with her as he explained about his different internet friends, his long-term interactions with them, and his social judgment in his online communications. His mother had a pleasant look on her face as she looked at him and attended to his story.

She remarked, "I never realized you had developed an online social life. I wish you hadn't kept those social interactions a secret. I was always so worried because I thought Jaylen was the only one you ever talk to."

James remained open with his mother about being Jamie. I recalled how he had explored his feminine side when he was playing as a child. I now understood more about his fascination with Rainbow Dash.

He shared this with his mother in another session. "I like dressing up as Jamie when I am alone in my room. I like when my online friends see me as her. I feel like I have been Jamie for a long time."

Arlene was learning more about his gender identity. "I like that you have your privacy in your room. I like that you have been able to share more about yourself with me. I feel sad that you have had to hide it."

When Arlene said this, I sensed that something had recently changed in their relationship. I saw a renewed sense of understanding between them in the way they now acknowledged each other.

Arlene asked him, "Would you like me to give you a dress to wear? I have some in the back of my closet that I never wear. I could show them to you. This would help you so you can look more like a girl when you see your friends online."

"Yes, that would be nice," he stated, as he grinned back at her. He seemed relieved. He was starting to feel understood.

After this, we talked more about his gender identity in treatment. James was now a high school senior. His mother had continued to be his educational advocate throughout high school. She had ensured accommodations were made for him to listen to audiobooks and read graphic novels for English. His writing had improved with the addition of using a word processor. To take notes in class, he was allowed to bring in his laptop, and he could take pictures of the assignments on the board with his phone. His father had gladly provided him with all the latest technological devices.

In treatment, James began to develop a better understanding of his gender identity. He said, "I liked female characters as a kid. When I played a character in a game, I wanted to play a female role. I think I have always been more secure with being female."

I encouraged him to see if he could explain this more. "I think I was assigned the wrong gender at birth," he told me. "The more I am Jamie, the better it makes me feel. Nobody at the high school knows me as Jamie. It's my secret. I can't wait to come home from school so I can be Jamie. When I'm in my room, I dress up, put on my makeup, and chat with my friends as Jamie."

James increasingly allowed his mother to become a part of his gender discovery. She accepted the changes. She helped provide him with a wardrobe that included clothes, jewelry, and makeup. She instructed him how to put on lipstick and blush and purchased bright dresses for him that he found on the internet. James identified as Jamie. He said he wanted to be Jamie even more.

He asked his mother during one of our sessions, "Could I dress up as Jamie for the whole weekend?"

Arlene said, "Why not?"

After several weekends of spending the entire time as Jamie, I wondered what the experience was like. "How did you feel dressing up as Jamie?" I asked.

"I feel so much more myself," he said. "I'm happier. I can't wait for the school week to end so I can be her."

He didn't talk much about his father, but I knew he still visited on weekends. I asked, "How does your father react to your outfits?"

He thought for a moment and responded with a half-smile. "You know, I don't think he even noticed. I wear a dress when we play computer games and at meals. He has never said anything."

James's sophistication with the internet gave him the means to research transgender issues. He became knowledgeable and began to establish goals for himself. He asserted to his mother and me that he wanted to transition to female. He had learned about the medical and psychological changes that he would have to undergo.

He said to us, "Could the two of you use the appropriate pronouns? Please refer to me as *she*, and as Jamie."

Arlene said, "I will try, but it may not be easy at first."

I agreed and said I would have to work on using the correct pronoun, too.

In a follow-up session, I went back to the subject of Jamie's dad. I expressed my concern that Ken was part of the family but didn't seem to have a clue about what was going on with Jamie. Jamie had said she wanted to explain to him her interest in transitioning. So I asked, "What does your father think?"

"I get no response from him," she said. She was disappointed, but was accustomed to her dad's usual slow reactions. "I decided to give him some transgender websites specifically for parents to look at."

I asked her again at a later time if her father was more understanding of her gender preference.

She shared, "It's taken him some time. My mother had to talk to him. But he's gotten better—he made a positive comment about my dress. The other day, he even said something about my hair. I haven't had to remind him to correct his pronouns. He has been referring to me as *she* and calling me Jamie. I think he is finally getting it." Jamie was pleased that her father had become more accepting of her.

* * *

Jamie felt accepted as female by her social media friends. Calvin, her closest internet friend, communicated daily with her through different messaging sources. She shared the most with him. She told Jaylen, her only high school friend, that she wanted to transition. Jamie had been a support to Jaylen as she was trying to understand her own sexuality. She shared with Jamie that she was pansexual.

I remember the first time Jamie came to her session as herself. She and her mother appeared nicely bonded like a mother and daughter sitting together in my waiting room. Arlene had on her usual shirt and pants outfit. Jamie, tall like her mother, wore a red-and-yellow-striped dress, and her hair was placed in a bun with a rainbow tie. She gave me a nice half-smile as I opened the door for her to come into my office. She sat on the couch with her legs crossed and looked right at me. Since this was her first public appearance, I asked, "How do you feel? You seem happy."

"I feel happier being Jamie," she said confidently. "I feel better in public. I don't mind if people look at me. I have been thinking about college. I want to wait to go until I can completely transition to Jamie. I want to start hormones, and medically become Jamie."

This was a new plan. She had already been accepted to several colleges.

"I want to enroll as Jamie. Which means I have to go through some medical procedures first," she said.

After Jamie graduated high school as James, Arlene continued to support her transition goal plan. Ken, meanwhile, had researched the medical procedure and went ahead and set up an appointment at a transgender clinic in a hospital facility.

Jamie was encouraged after her visit to the clinic. Arlene said they needed a letter from me so the insurance would cover the medical treatment. I said I would summarize her treatment history with me, her psychological transition from male to female, and her commitment to continue to confirm her female identity through hormones and gender-affirming surgery. Before I sent the letter, I would need Jamie's consent to release it.

I noticed that Arlene appeared edgy and sat on the couch next to Jamie with her hands tightly clasped together. She wouldn't look at me or Jamie. She seemed to be bothered by some other concern. I asked her, "Are you worried about something?"

Arlene said, "Do you think Jamie is still on the autism spectrum? She seems so different—more sensitive, more social, and even empathic. She asked me the other day how she can help around the house! In the past, she never cared or noticed."

I explained to the both of them my understanding of autism. I said that Jamie would always have characteristics of autism, such as rigid, fixated approaches and social limitations, but these differences shouldn't inhibit her choices. "She has found that the more she expresses herself as Jamie the more confident she becomes," I said. "She realizes that she can only handle one task at a time; therefore, she wants to complete her medical transition before going to college. Socially, she has learned she was more comfortable communicating online than in person. Jamie, I believe, is able to accept her autism, and she appears to be doing the best she can with it."

Both of them agreed. The session ended.

* * *

Jamie began her medical transition. I was able to observe the maturing of her feminine side as the hormones changed her physical appearance. Jamie would come to her sessions wearing one of the many different outfits she had picked out for herself. Arlene had had her hair styled at a salon. The hormones reduced her facial hair, and her body was developing gradually to appear more feminine.

In one of our sessions, she sat on her favorite area on the left side of the couch in my office and pointed her long, thin fingers to show me her colored nails. She said, "They represent the colors of the rainbow. I did them myself. Do you remember how I always liked Rainbow Dash? I was thinking about her when I colored them."

I said, "You introduced me to Rainbow Dash when we first met. You told me you wanted to be her."

She talked about how much had changed since then. "I feel more like a girl. People refer to me as *she*. An older man held the door open for me. I feel more accepted as female. I am legally going to change my name to Jamie."

I pointed out that she appeared to move the area around her mouth more, which resulted in her expressing a complete smile. I had never seen her do this before, and it helped her show more feeling. I was curious if she was aware of the difference in her smile.

She said, "Thank you! I look in the mirror and practice different facial expressions. I like seeing myself as female. I even work on the sound of my voice. Seeing and listening to myself helps me feel more like I am Jamie."

She liked the way the hormones made her feel. She shaved the hair on her legs and under her arms. I noticed her skin appeared smooth and softer.

She went on, "I can't deal with having a penis. It annoys me. I can't hide it. I think I want to have the vaginoplasty surgery."

In the next session, Jamie said she had committed to having her surgery at the hospital associated with the transgender clinic she had been attending. Her mother, who was present, supported her decision. I asked about her other supports.

She gave her mother that full smile she had been working on and said, "I have both my parents and especially my mom to be there for me. I have Calvin, too. We talk all the time and have become close. He knows about my surgery and says he will be there for me. Someday we hope to meet."

I attempted to engage her in discussing pain management and other aspects about the medical procedure, but she wasn't interested. She only thought about the outcome—of beginning her life as Jamie. Jamie and Arlene attended treatment until close to the scheduled surgery. I then transferred her treatment to a counselor at the clinic who was specially trained in pre- and post-surgery interventions. After Jamie had fully recovered from the procedure, Arlene contacted me at a later time to tell me that Jamie had started a computer science program and was living in a women's dorm at college.

I will always remember Jamie's termination statement in our last session before her surgery. She said, "Thank you for helping me become myself. I will never forget how you let me bring Rainbow Dash to my sessions. I stopped collecting the figures. I can't wait to complete the surgery. It will be a new beginning for me. Being Jamie will be something I can't finish. I will have to keep working on being Jamie."

CHALLENGES AND REFLECTIONS

Arlene introduced me to the family by explaining their story in our intake session. I had never met Ken, James's father. Arlene had caring feelings for Ken but had difficulties with his cumbersome social interactions. I could see that she worried about James being too much like his father. James liked our play therapy interactions. He enjoyed gender creative play themes. He learned communication skills through his stories. James was persistent to confirm her gender identity. She wanted to become Jamie. This intention pulled the family together in our treatment.

In the beginning of therapy, James was a challenge to engage. He was not an easy child to connect with and form a relationship. He made no eye contact, he had odd mannerisms, and he tended to avoid my usual attempts to socially interact with him. I knew he was on the autism spectrum. I could see that a therapeutic relationship with him would have its difficulties. I had to think outside the box. When he reluctantly came into my therapy office he didn't acknowledge my toys or games as most other children would have. I observed that his limited conversation centered on his favorite pony, Rainbow Dash. In order to appeal to him, I would have to accept what interested him. I let him introduce me into his play culture. He would have to tell me about why he liked My Little Pony characters. I listened to him. I needed to understand and learn about his world. This type of interaction was what helped develop our therapeutic relationship. He eventually enjoyed making up play stories with his special toy figures. He allowed me into his inner play culture. By understanding his unique interests, I was able to form a closer bond with him. I expanded on his play interests. I worked them into our treatment to improve his communication skills. He valued our therapeutic interaction.

The trust that James and I had built helped him feel safe in telling me about his gender explorations. He told me about his special online long-term friendships. James shared with me how he wanted to transition to Jamie in treatment. I accepted that her adolescent path fit into her other childhood behavior patterns that I observed. I followed her lead and offered her support. She asked me and her mother to change pronouns from *he/him* to *she/her*. I recognized how important this was to her. Arlene and I made the effort to identify her as Jamie and use the proper pronouns during our sessions.

In family treatment, Jamie explained to her mother Arlene her wish to transition. Arlene was Jamie's advocate. She supported her decision to go through a medical transition. It was a challenge to get Ken, her father, to come to one of our sessions. Ken was brought into Jamie's personal decision by Arlene and Jamie.

In order for Jamie to participate in treatment, Arlene had to be invested from the beginning. She was her primary caregiver. I had to establish a therapeutic relationship with her. I developed a way to connect with her by helping her learn about Jamie's autism. Instead of me being the one to insist on the autism diagnosis, I worked with her. We discovered it together. In time as Arlene understood the pattern of Jamie's behavior, the better she was able to parent her.

Arlene remained supportive of Jamie throughout our therapy. She became her most important support when she transitioned from James to Jamie during our treatment. She helped in getting Ken to accept Jamie's changes. A challenge of my therapy with Jamie was to know when our treatment was over. When would she require something different? This happened when she needed to go to a counselor with a specialty in transgender issues and pre- and post-surgery care.

Chapter 3

Angry Dan

PRESENTING PROBLEMS

Dan was brought into treatment by his mother, Beth. He was five years old. Beth was worried. Dan seemed to be an angry boy. He would hit his peers and throw his toys. Dan had witnessed significant domestic assaults between her and his father, Larry, since he was an infant. She reported that the incidents of physical aggression escalated with Larry's drinking. After Dan witnessed a severe fight between his parents, Beth had decided to call the police. She was done with Larry. She wanted Dan to get help. She was concerned that he would be violent like his father.

Dan's treatment began with play therapy interventions to help with his aggressive actions. He needed to learn caring responses. His therapy continued through his adolescence. He learned cognitive behavioral strategies to manage his anger. As a teenager, he developed empathy in his relationships. Dan found some relief. He showed sensitivity and respect for women. He believed he had his substance use under control.

Dan's relationship with his father, Larry, was problematic. When Dan would stay at Larry's household as a teenager, Larry would often drink excessively. This usually ended up with Dan and his father having an argument and a loud, angry encounter. Dan completed treatment near the end of high school. I hoped he would be successful in managing his anger and in control of his substance use.

I was surprised when I found out he was incarcerated. He assaulted someone while intoxicated. Dan's legal situation resulted in Dan being ordered into a specialized substance abuse program. Even though he wasn't in treatment with me anymore I learned that he had benefited from our long-term therapeutic relationship.

TREATMENT STORY

The phone call from Dan's mother had troubled me from the beginning. "He can't control his anger!" she said to me. "I don't want him to be like his father. His father is in jail. He was drunk and beat me up in front of the boy. I had had it. I called the police on him."

She continued and said, "I am worried because Dan is only five years old, but he has seen so much of our fighting. He's been throwing toys and hitting his peers at school. Maggie, his teacher, told me he needs help."

I gave her a time to come in alone. I wanted to understand from her perspective what the child had witnessed. How much violence had he seen? What was his relationship with his father like?

Beth was a stocky woman with strong facial features, short, light-colored hair, and a pained look on her face. She followed me directly into my office and began talking immediately. She didn't even give me a chance to sit down.

"It started right after the baby was born," she began. "Larry seemed to always be mad. It was like he didn't want to be a father. He refused to hold the baby or change his diapers. I had to do everything." She continued almost without a breath: "He would call me stupid, an idiot, and complained I could never do anything right. When the baby cried, he yelled at me and told me to shut the kid up. He acted like he was my boss."

I realized I would have to slow down her pace, so I asked her questions about Larry's behavior. "Did Larry help you in any way with Dan? What did you do with Dan when the two of you were fighting?" I asked.

"It was me who made sure the baby was up to date on his shots. I was his main caretaker," she said. "I did my best to keep Dan away from the arguing. I would take him with me into his room and stay with him. Larry would leave us alone in there."

"Can you tell me more about the extent of Larry's drinking?"

"It got worse over time," she said. "The more he drank, the meaner he became. Things about the baby upset him. He couldn't take it when Dan whined, cried, or needed attention. This seemed to make him drink more!"

I suspected Larry was an alcoholic. I wondered if he used alcohol as self-medication for an underlying emotional problem. It appeared that having a family seemed to exacerbate his drinking. "Why do you think Larry drank?"

"Larry's father was a severe alcoholic," Beth said. "Larry told me he beat his mother and left him when he was a small child. I don't know. Maybe he resented not having his own father."

"How did Larry end up incarcerated?" I asked. This had occurred several months before she contacted me. I hoped she would be willing to explain the incident to me.

She said, "He had been drinking a lot. He was upset about his job. A coworker who started several months after he did got a promotion and was now his boss. He was angry and said it wasn't fair. He thought he was a better worker. Dan was sitting with us on the couch while we were watching a football game. He accidentally knocked over Larry's beer can as he crawled onto my lap, and Larry lost it. He punched me. Dan ran into his room. I went in to see if he was okay. He was hiding in the closet, crying. I couldn't take it anymore. I stayed with him, as I usually did."

She had calmed down since she first came into the office and seemed relieved telling me about the incident. She appeared less tense. I believe she felt she had done the right thing by protecting and comforting her child. But she was definitely bothered by what happened. I wondered why she said she had had it with Larry. I asked her, "What was different this time?"

"He hit me!" she said. "He was drunk as usual, and he put his hands on me. I had told him when he slapped me a couple of months ago if he ever did it again, I was done. This was the last straw. I sat with Dan in his bedroom closet, holding him, and I called the police on my cell phone. When I let the officers in, Larry was passed out. I had a bruise on my face and was still holding on to Dan. When Larry saw them, he jumped up and went after me. The officers had to physically remove him from our apartment," she said.

The boy certainly had witnessed physical aggression, I said to her. I was not surprised he had anger issues. I asked, "Besides his teacher, has anyone else complained about his behavior?"

"Yes, my mother has," she said. "Meme, as Dan calls her, watches him. I have to work some Saturdays, so she takes him for the day. She told me he smashed a toy truck she had bought him."

"Did your mother tell you *why* Dan destroyed the truck?" I asked. I was hoping to get a better picture of Dan's angry reactions.

She said, "My mother said she thought he loved that toy truck. He would always play with it. She thought it was one of his favorite toys. So she was completely surprised by his behavior. All she had done was ask him to put his things away. He grabbed the truck and threw it against the wall and broke it."

I asked, "Did your mother notice anything else that day about Dan that might have caused him to act in such a way?"

She said, "She just said he might have been tired. She hadn't given him lunch yet, and she was rushing him to get things picked up."

I thanked her for the background information she shared and told her that we could target Dan's anger as a treatment goal. I explained to her that she would be part of the therapy. She would have the important role of providing me with feedback about his behavior. This would be helpful so I could monitor his progress on learning to manage his anger.

She consented to bring the boy in for the next appointment.

* * *

The following week, Dan sat next to his mother in the waiting area. The boy was broad and heavily built like his mother. He was neatly dressed. When I introduced myself, he looked at me with some trepidation. He stayed close to his mother as they came into my office.

"Look at the toys," his mother said as she pointed them out. Dan seemed to feel more at ease as he scanned the play items in my office.

I told Dan how children liked coming into my office to play with the different toys and games. Dan walked to the shelf next to the couch and grabbed a tin filled with army men off it. His mother watched, not knowing what to do.

His aggressiveness in taking something in a new place without asking—and his mother's lack of response—concerned me. I wondered if this was Dan's attempt to control the situation. I realized his impulsivity would have to be addressed, and I decided it was important for me to immediately add structure and boundaries to the play.

"Would you like to play with the army men?" I said calmly. He haphazardly dumped the figures out of the bin on top of the child's table.

I said, "We can play with them together while your mother goes back out to the waiting room."

He seemed to trust the idea of playing something with me. "Okay!" he blurted. He watched as I opened my office door for his mother to leave.

I tried to set up a structured play scenario. I said, "We can have some fun with the army men. Let's play with them at the sand table." I scooped the army figures back into the tin. I lifted up the table cover and shoved it behind the multipurpose table next to the wall. It was now ready for sand play. I placed the tin on top of the sand. I said, "Let's each take some army men and place them in the sand."

Instead of strategically positioning them like I started doing, he grabbed the army men and threw them into the sand. His sudden actions were difficult to anticipate. I smiled at him. "Please don't throw them. Be kind to my army men."

He responded, "Okay."

I slowly arranged the small soldiers on wooden blocks I had put in the sand. He observed my actions. He was interested. "These are barracks," I said to him. I asked if he wanted the green or brown team.

"I want these guys," he said as he sorted out a handful of green soldiers.

We created two different factions based on color. I was hoping this fine-motor exercise would focus his actions. It did.

Dan commented, "There always has to be good and bad guys."

As we were carefully organizing our teams, I decided to see how he would respond to a question about his father. "Why didn't your dad come today?" I was not entirely surprised by his reaction. He immediately tossed the empty container into the edge of the sand table.

He stated, "My daddy is in jail! He hit my mommy!"

"I'm sorry to hear that," I said. I decided directly talking about his father was too sensitive an issue for him to process at this time. I realized it was best to go back to playing.

I said, "Angry soldiers who can't learn to control their temper end up in an army jail." I put some blocks in the corner and said to him, "This could be the jail." Then, in an effort to get him to contribute to the structured activity, I said, "How many men should we each have on our team?"

We both picked up the figures he scattered, so we could set up our spaces. As he touched each of his small, green toy soldiers he counted, "One, two, three, four, five." He was pleased to demonstrate his counting ability and provide me with an answer. "Five!" he said.

We played in parallel. We each continued to separate out the army men according to color. We each positioned the soldiers on the wooden block structures, pretending they were army barracks. I noticed his tongue protruded out of the right side of his mouth as he offered a cheeky smile. He appeared visibly relieved to manipulate and set up the pieces and not talk about his father. I was pleased to see him being able to enjoy our cooperative fun. When the scene was completed, I said to him, "We should let your mother in to show her what you made."

Dan said, "Let's show Mommy. I'll get her."

Before I had a chance to respond, he darted out the door into the waiting area. His mother followed him back in. He was excited to show her what he had made.

"See what I did?" he said as he pointed to the sand table.

His mother observed the ordered army figures. While she eyed the figures, he began destroying the scene we had just made with thrashing hand chops. Beth didn't know how to respond. She just stood there with that same pained look on her face I had noticed earlier.

Looking to me now, she said, "This is what he does at home! His toys are all over the place and broken. When I ask him to put things away, he gets mad and throws stuff. He makes me so upset."

I said to her, "You need a response to his behavior."

I began moving the disarrayed toy soldiers into piles. He helped. I asked him to tell me where his safest and favorite spot was in their apartment. He said, "My room."

I suggested she might want to use a simple counting parenting procedure to counter his actions. I said, "This can help him think about his behavior and act as a consequence if he doesn't listen." She could use his room as a safe, calming space for him. Dan listened intently to our conversation.

He and his mother agreed that his room could be his special safe space when he needed a break. I explained to him that his mother would help him decide when he needed calming time. She would do this by counting 1-2-3. "Let's practice," I said. I placed a truck on the floor. I smiled at Dan and said, "Let's pretend Dan refuses to pick up this truck." I looked at Beth and told her to begin counting. I encouraged her to remind Dan after each number what she wanted him to do. This would allow him a chance to remediate his behavior.

She smiled at Dan, raised a finger, and said, "One! You need to pick up your truck." She added a second finger and said, "Two! Please pick up your truck, or you will have to go to your room." After raising one more finger, she said, "Three! This is the last time I will ask. If you don't pick up your truck you will have to go to your room."

The boy listened to his mother count. He carefully watched as she put her fingers up. He seemed so engrossed in the exercise that he automatically responded with, "Okay, Mommy!"

Beth liked the parenting plan. Dan assisted me in putting back the items we had played with. As we were putting things away, he said, "Can we play with them again?" I gave them another appointment.

In the next set of sessions, I addressed more of Dan's angry reactions. When he was impulsive, I became quicker to intervene. For instance, when he would attempt to grab the toys off the shelf, I would counter his actions by instructing him to use words and ask me for what he wanted.

In order to mediate his aggressive actions, I also added more thought-out play activities. I did this by introducing a different theme to our army game. I advocated for the idea that we had to describe the skills and training our fighters had. I showed him an example by taking one of my soldiers and had that soldier leap through the air over to his side. I said he had developed this special skill to be a good soldier.

He said, "Like the Teenage Mutant Ninja Turtles."

"That's right!" I said. "Master Splinter trained the Teenage Mutant Ninja Turtles for many, many years, so they had skills to help society." Dan nodded in agreement. After we finished developing our respective army bases, I showed him how to add action rules. I had my specially trained soldier leap over to Dan's side, jump on one of his soldiers, and knock the soldier down. He seemed intrigued by including this type of activity to our play.

I proposed doing the game of "Rock, Paper, Scissors" to see who goes first. He agreed, and we counted to three and showed our hands.

"I won!" he said, and showed me how his two fingers formed a pair of scissors that could cut my flat hand, which represented a piece of paper. He would get to go first. I reminded him that we would be taking turns.

He learned over time to follow the rules I set up for our playtime. He would often test me, but I reminded him that we wouldn't be able to continue playing unless he followed the rules. As the weeks went on, I expanded our play by introducing more cooperative and empathic interactions. I expected these treatment goals to further help calm his antagonistic reactions. I did this through persuading Dan to allow our army teams to work together and fight for the common good. Eventually, he became comfortable enough to play alone while I went out to get his mother in the waiting room.

His mother became experienced at providing me with regular feedback on his progress. She reported that my therapeutic interventions were translating into Dan having more patience and better self-control at home. The parenting strategies I taught her, including counting to three and sending Dan to his room, were working well. Dan lost his temper less frequently, and he often played by himself in his room. "He doesn't seem as angry," she told me.

* * *

It was about a year and a half later that Beth brought up a new concern.

"Larry has been released from jail," she told me during a family session in my office. "He is demanding to see Dan."

Dan, who had been playing with some toy vehicles in the sand, turned around from the table and looked at me and his mother. "Do I have to see him?"

Instead of answering her son, Beth continued talking to me. "Larry made no effort to contact Dan during his jail time. He gave me full custody. I don't know what to do. I don't think he's changed!"

I said, "It seems like you're worried about Dan's safety. Since you have full custody, you can request supervised visits. In this way, the interactions between Dan and his father can be monitored by a trained caseworker." She liked my suggestion and said she would contact the court and check it out.

* * *

I had a session with Dan shortly after his first supervised visit with his father. He was now in first grade. I approached him in the waiting area where he was sitting next to his mother. He had a scowl on his face. He didn't greet me or look at me. His mother stood as I came over, her mouth and jaw tight with anguish, and said, "He was so upset after he saw his father, he came home and threw his things all over his room."

I smiled at Dan and tried to engage him: "Would you like to come in and play with the toys in my office?"

He struggled to return the smile and said, "The army men?"

In my office, we sat next to each other. We set up our teams of soldiers in a similar manner as we had done before in earlier sessions. As we arranged our small characters, I excitedly introduced a new theme. "What if we join forces and see if we can defeat the mean monster that was destroying society?" I pulled down from the toy shelf a Gila-like creature with numerous protruding plastic teeth. I held up the figure to show him and entice his interest. "This will be the beast," I said to him.

He nodded his head in agreement, and in his enthusiasm for playing with me, he stated, "Let's build a cave for the monster."

Playing in tandem, we constructed a wooden area for the toy demon. We surrounded the aggressive-looking creature with our soldiers. I said, "Let's capture and tame the destructive beast." We pretended to make the sounds of guns firing. I pushed the figure down in the sand. "We did it! The beast has been tamed!" I was pleased to say. "We're a good team!"

He was pleased by our accomplishment as well. "Yes, we did it!" he said.

I said, "You know that your mother said she didn't like that you threw your toys all over your room after seeing your father."

He said, "I know."

I said, "Your father has been in jail for being mean and angry. Maybe like the beast we just tamed, your father might have learned not to be so mad." I asked him if anything good happened at the visit.

The boy had been listening carefully to me and said, "He showed me how to play war with cards. He was nice."

I took out a deck of cards, and he showed me how to play the game of war. Later, Beth came into the session, and I proposed that she have a safety plan in place for after the visits. I advised her that she might want to put limited demands on Dan. I suggested she allow him to deescalate; maybe she could get him something to eat or let him play quietly in his room after seeing his father.

Over time, the boy's relationship with his father did improve. Supervision was discontinued, and his father was able to obtain a legal visitation schedule.

By the time Larry was nearing the end of his probationary period, I had been seeing Dan for about three years. Larry had moved into an apartment with his girlfriend, Jean. She had two children: John was eight, the same age as Dan, and Marilyn was about seven. Larry shared this information one day when he contacted me to arrange an appointment. The stated purpose was for him to learn about his son's problems so he could better parent him. He said to me he was asking the court for overnights every other weekend.

Beth was hesitant and suspicious, but she accepted that it was important for Larry to come in and meet with me about his son. She said, "I don't trust Larry. I think he is up to something. He is asking the court for overnights. He probably doesn't want to pay so much child support. Maybe you will see for yourself when you meet with him. I guess it has to happen. He is the father."

I explained to Larry when I spoke with him on the phone that I would have to tell Dan of our conversation. I wanted to let the boy know what I would discuss and how I would protect his privacy. The boy seemed hopeful when

I told him I was going to meet with his father. Dan said, "Tell him to do stuff with me when I come over."

At this time, Dan was not only adjusting to his father's new relationship, but his mother was involved with someone as well. After seeing Bill for a while, she had moved into Bill's doublewide trailer. His six-year-old son, Steven, had consistent weekly overnight visits. Bill worked in a manufacturing plant. Beth appreciated the way Bill played ball with both boys. She told me that Bill was a calm, relaxed person. She enjoyed the way he responded to her child.

Dan continued to make progress on his angry reactions. He said to me in one of our sessions, "When I get mad, I can now walk away." This was a strategy we had discussed in our therapy.

This was the current situation of Dan's life when his father came in to meet with me. Larry, a tall, thin man with a ruddy look on his face, attempted to stare me down as I came into the waiting room to get him. "Are you Dan's father, Larry?" I politely asked.

"So you are the counselor I hear about!" he said gruffly.

"Would you like to come into my office so we could talk about Dan, privately?" I was trying to be nice and made an effort to engage him. "I was hoping you could share some of your thoughts about him."

As soon as he sat down in my office, I could tell this may not happen. He continued to glare at me as he placed himself in the chair and solidly planted his feet on the floor. I could tell he was bothered by meeting with me. I guessed that he felt forced to do so in order to establish that he was a good father and help get the overnights he wanted with his son.

"It was her fault!" he said. "I wouldn't be in this mess if it wasn't for her. I wanted to work it out, but she had to involve the police! I know no matter what I say to you, you will be on her side."

He already had a preconceived judgment, so I tried to reframe our interaction. I proposed, "I am your son's therapist. We should talk about him." To be extra clear, I added, "The purpose of us meeting today isn't to work on your relationship with Beth. I was hoping we could talk about your and Dan's relationship."

He said, "He wants to be with me. I'm his father. He says he wants to live with me. I know what's best for him!"

I knew this wasn't an accurate statement about Dan's preferences. I decided my best approach was to be straight with him. I brought up the observations that were reported to me by the caseworker supervising his interactions with his son. I said, "The caseworker reported to me that she had concerns about you being critical and loud with Dan when she observed your interactions with him." I said, "She believed from her observations that Dan was upset by your actions. I asked her if she tried to explain this to you. She said she tried, but you refused to listen."

Larry's hands and arms tensed, and he continued to glare at me. With a loud voice, he complained, "The ladies watching those visits don't know what they're talking about! They told me they thought my son was afraid of me. They don't know anything. He's my son!"

I started to respond with a question, but he interrupted me. He was upset. "Listen to me!" he demanded. "I never knew my father. He was a drunk. He beat my mother. He left when I was little. I never saw him again. That won't happen with my son. I am going to see him no matter what his mother says or does."

"I'm sorry about your father," I said. "I realize you don't want this for your son." I tried again to help him understand what his son was dealing with. "Dan is trying to manage his own anger, and I was hoping you could help him with this."

"That's because his mother is forcing that guy Bill on him," Larry shot back. "She wants him to be the father. That won't happen!"

I tried again to empathize with him. I said, "Your son just wants to have a good relationship with you. Beth wants that, too. The boy needs you as much as his mother."

"I know the boy needs a father," he said. Then in the next breath he insisted, "I have every right to see my son! I'm done talking with you! You can't tell me how to talk to my son!"

The session didn't end well. I was not sure if I was able to help him understand any of his son's concerns. He left my office just as angry as he was when he came in. He refused to accept responsibility for his behavior or Dan's anger. He believed he was not at fault. He believed Beth was doing everything she could to keep him away from his son. I was disappointed that I couldn't engage Larry to be part of Dan's treatment.

I discussed my meeting with Larry with Dan and his mother the next time they came in. Beth was not surprised by Larry's behavior. She didn't think Larry understood the purpose of Dan's therapy. She felt that Larry didn't realize how his mean, nasty, and angry reactions affected his son. We all agreed that Dan would have to do his best to adapt to the legally mandated visits. He liked his father's girlfriend and got along well with her son, John. They often played video games together. These relationships would provide some support for him when at Larry's home.

In time, Dan adjusted to having his father back in his life again. He managed to deal with his father by avoiding him. His father worked third shift and wasn't around when Dan was at his home for overnight visits. When he came in for our therapy sessions during his middle school years, he usually talked about his peer group, not about his father. He shared with me his interest in having a girlfriend—someone he could get along with and not argue with. Even though I didn't see him as frequently as I did in the past, he had fond memories of those early playtimes.

Once I asked him how he was managing his anger now that he was a teenager. He pointed to the Gila-like creature on my shelf and said, "I'm like that beast we tamed." He truly seemed to have a better handle on his anger. He graduated the eighth grade, and we discontinued therapy for a period of time.

* * *

I hadn't seen Dan for more than a year when Beth contacted me. She was upset. She told me on the phone that Dan seemed to be angry again. "He says high school is annoying," Beth said. "He gets irritated when Bill or I ask him to do something. We just had a big fight the other night. He told Bill that he's not his father, and he doesn't have to listen to him. I got mad! I told him he should go live with his father. After things calmed down, we agreed it would be good for him to talk to you."

I could tell Dan was reluctant to meet with me as soon as I saw him in the waiting room. He was sitting on the opposite side of the room from his mother. He had grown to be a sturdy-looking adolescent. He didn't look at his mother or me when I came out to get him. He came into the office and flopped onto the couch without a word. I knew I had to gain his attention, and I decided that addressing the argument with his mother wasn't the way to start. Instead, I asked him, "Have you thought about what kind of work you would like to do?"

I was right, he hadn't been expecting this and was comfortable answering my question. He said, "My friends work at fast-food places. I don't know what I want to do. I need a skill. I don't like school. I heard about a police program at the high school. The cops around here have a nice car and house."

I said that I knew several other teenagers who completed the law enforcement curriculum at the high school. I said that it was an excellent way to move into police work or other similar jobs. Talking about a work plan and his independence instead of the conflicts at home seemed to engage him. I offered him the option of coming into therapy on a monthly basis to explore his future options.

At the end of our session, he said, "I know my mother wants the best for me. I know I could never live with my father." I scheduled another appointment with his mother so she could transport him. She respected his privacy and didn't ask me what we talked about in our session.

Over the next couple of years, Dan continued to attend therapy. His mother always brought him, and sometimes I would briefly inform her of Dan's progress with his permission. Dan moved toward more independence; he obtained a part-time job, got his driver's license, and was accepted into the law enforcement program at the high school. A teacher at the program was one of the officers who helped his mother out with his father. The two of them formed a positive bond.

Dan made a connection between school and work. The idea of police work sparked his interest. He could help others and have a decent life—a theme, I reminded him, that we had played out at the sand table with the soldiers when he was a child. He said, "I like police shows. My mother and Bill sometimes watch them with me."

His home life, at this time, was becoming more chaotic. He didn't like staying at his mother's because she had too many rules. He told her that he was staying at his father's. "Really," he said to me, "I'm at my girlfriend Emma's house every night."

Dan shared with me his insight about his parents. "My mother has always been there for me. I think when I was a kid, I wanted to be home to protect her. But she worries too much. My father, I don't know if he is even capable of caring about me."

I reminded him that his mother first brought him in because she didn't want him to follow in his father's footsteps.

He said, "I don't want alcohol to mess up my life. My father can't stop drinking. He drinks all the time. He yelled at me to get a job. I then got a job. He told me I need to pay rent. I just stay away from him."

Because of the history of addiction on his father's side, I was worried about Dan's potential for substance abuse. When I told him that, he had an answer.

"I limit my partying," he said. "Sure, I drink, and do some drugs, but I try to be careful. In my mind, I keep the memory of what drinking did to my father and mother. I say to myself drinking is my father's problem."

Several months before Dan would graduate from high school, we had our final meeting. He had continued therapy but was ready to finish. I asked him if he would like to reflect on our time together. I especially wanted to see if he understood the pattern of anger and alcoholism and how it can affect a relationship.

He told me that he had made important life commitments so he wouldn't repeat his parents' mistakes. He said, "I'm mostly at Emma's house. She helps me like my mother did. She's going into nursing, and I'm going into criminal justice at the same community college. I like her parents. They don't drink or fight. They're good to me."

Dan left me with hope for his success. He had worked hard at controlling his anger, and he wanted to improve his life. He recognized the problems of violence and alcoholism in his family. I was impressed that he had established a respectful relationship with Emma and her family. He was about to complete the law enforcement program at the high school. I wished him well.

* * *

I thought I had closed Dan's case. But in the fall, I was contacted by a forensic psychologist, Dr. Held. I knew Dr. Held because we had spoken in the past about cases we had in common. He did risk assessments for the state when a legal determination needed to be made about the benefit of treatment or further incarceration. He had obtained a release from Dan to talk with me. The release asked me to share clinical information about Dan's treatment. The summary on the paperwork said that Dan had been incarcerated due to being charged with assault. Dr. Held was assessing Dan to determine his risk of harming others and committing further violent acts. He had questions for me about Dan's treatment as a factor in establishing sentencing and his risk to harm.

Dr. Held examined risk factors such as a teenager's history of violence, learning issues, family discord, and substance abuse. But he also assessed protective factors like anger management strategies, self-control, prosocial behaviors, and commitment to therapy. This was why Dr. Held wanted to learn about Dan's engagement in therapy. I, too, had some questions for Dr. Held. I wondered about what had precipitated the incident. I knew it was not like Dan to be violent. Something unusual must have happened. Dr. Held and I set up a time to talk on the phone as part of his evaluation. I asked him what had happened.

Dr. Held said, "Dan was at a party with his friends and was significantly intoxicated. Another individual got into an argument with Dan's girlfriend. Loud words were exchanged, and this individual pushed his girlfriend and slammed her to the ground. She screamed for him to get away from her. Dan attacked the guy."

I asked Dr. Held if he had interviewed Dan about the incident. He said he did. I wondered if he was able to tell me what Dan told him about what had happened.

Dr. Held said, "Dan told me he had been quite angry before the party. He said he and his father had a fight. His father pushed him. He knew his father was drunk. He had enough sense to leave his father's house, and then went to the party. The individual who caused harm to his girlfriend was an old boyfriend of hers. He told me he never liked him. The boy had been abusive to her. Dan admitted he had been drinking heavily. He said when he heard his girlfriend screaming, he completely lost control. He said he might have blacked out. He had limited recollection of what happened." Dan was charged with assault because the other individual was hospitalized with a broken jaw and head injuries. He was unconscious and had to be transported to the emergency room. Observers said it took several of his friends to pull Dan away from him.

I described for Dr. Held Dan's early history, the abuse he witnessed, and his father's alcoholism. I reviewed the course of his therapy and how Dan struggled with his anger and aggression. I said he never had any assaultive incidents when I worked with him. And I informed Dr. Held about Dan's conflicted relationship with his father and how he tried to make it better.

Dr. Held asked, "Was substance abuse dealt with in his treatment?"

I said that we talked about his vulnerability to addiction, but it was toward the end of treatment. Dan told me he didn't want substance abuse to be part of his life and affect his relationships. I explained to Dr. Held that I didn't specifically focus on alcoholism. I had addressed his anger and the need to learn to respect others.

I had a long-term relationship with Dan and cared about him. I was aware that Dr. Held's recommendations would have an impact on his future. I knew Dr. Held always took account of how amenable someone was to therapy. I asked him if he had formulated any conclusions.

Dr. Held said, "I believe that Dan's most significant risk factor was witnessing the violence from his father as a child. His drinking as a teenager certainly disinhibited him and probably exacerbated his assaulting someone else who was being overly aggressive to someone he also cared about. I do not plan to designate him as a person who is at high risk of harming others. Since Dan benefited from therapy, I will recommend a specialized sentence. This would include a substance abuse program for him and treatment as an alternative to further incarceration."

I knew Dr. Held was right that Dan could benefit from a substance abuse treatment program. But I also believed that Dr. Held respected Dan's ongoing efforts to better himself and engage in therapy. I had watched Dan deal with an angry, alcoholic father figure and work hard in his treatment not to repeat the same pattern. I knew Dr. Held saw Dan as I did: not as someone who was at risk of harming others, but as someone who wanted to help others and himself. I felt some hope for Dan in the future and believed that Dr. Held's giving him a second chance could make a difference.

CHALLENGES AND REFLECTIONS

Dan's experience of violence remained a theme throughout the stages of his development. It was clearly expressed in his play. His mother's support helped. Dan struggled to control his anger. He worked hard at not being like his father. He recognized that his father was demeaning and critical of him. Dan didn't recognize how the use of substances affected his ability to manage his anger.

Teaching young children to manage their anger and aggression is a therapeutic challenge. Dan witnessed and experienced violent behavior for many years from his father before he began treatment. As a young child, Dan enjoyed play therapy. He liked to set up the army figures and have pretend play battles. I encouraged him to describe the fighting. He talked about the aggressive actions his figures engaged in within our play therapy sessions. This helped him think about his actions. I then introduced cooperative, empathic, and nonviolent responses into our play treatment. In time, as a young child Dan began to understand the differences between cooperative and aggressive responses. This translated into his improved behavior at home and in school. Beth had been a supportive and caring parent. She established consistent rules at home. She intervened when he became aggressive.

Dan had a difficult time managing his anger when he was a teenager. This was complicated because of his conflictual interactions with his father. Larry wasn't supportive of him. Larry was demanding and controlling. Dan saw that his father had a significant alcohol abuse problem. His parents each had legal rights. The divorce split between the household resulted in Dan getting mixed messages. He had two different sets of rules. I attempted to establish some kind of parental consistency. Larry stated he knew better. He refused to participate in the intervention.

Another challenge I had to deal with was Dan's substance abuse. As a teenager, Dan used substances with his peers. He believed he had control of his alcohol use. I thought he did, too. He said he wasn't like his father. Dan and I were wrong. Dan became involved with the legal system after we terminated our treatment. His overuse of alcohol and drugs resulted in him having a violent encounter.

I learned about Dan's dangerous and aggressive actions from Dr. Held, a forensic evaluator. I advocated for Dan in talking with Dr. Held. This was an important part of my therapeutic relationship with Dan. I wanted to convey to Dr. Held that Dan struggled in therapy to change his pattern of anger. In evaluating Dan's violence risk, Dr. Held took into account what Dan gained from our long-term therapy relationship. Through our conversations, Dr. Held became aware of Dan's past attempts to correct his behavior. I believe this prompted Dr. Held to suggest that Dan be court ordered to participate in a substance abuse program instead of going to jail.

Chapter 4

The Trauma Binder

PRESENTING PROBLEMS

Peggy organized the details of her grandchildren's early trauma experience in a binder. In our intake session, she shared this information. She wanted Jasmine, who was five and a half, and Javon, who was four, seen for therapy. They were neglected and suffered abuse in their mother Joan's home. The booklet helped Peggy put the incidents into perspective.

Peggy and Harold, their step-grandfather, provided the children with a stable and safe home environment. They were taken away from Joan. She was Peggy's daughter and a severe drug addict. She was legally deemed unable to care for her children.

Peggy consistently brought Jasmine and Javon in for treatment. The treatment was long term. Each child dealt with the effects that early trauma had on their childhood and adolescence. By participating in their grandchildren's treatment, Peggy and Harold learned how trauma was an integral part of their development. In their late adolescence, their grandparents were supportive when Jasmine and Javon wanted to distance themselves from their mother.

This case involved two children in the same family who needed treatment. Ruth and I worked together on the case. We had a similar treatment approach to the problem. Ruth and I agreed that trauma had a developmental effect on children. Our co-therapy involved combining system issues, cognitive-behavioral strategies, and calming techniques.

TREATMENT STORY

Jasmine and Javon were children whose experience of trauma defined their psychological makeup. Peggy, their maternal grandmother, contacted me

51

asking for help when Jasmine was about five and a half, and Javon was almost four. She sounded quite worried and overwhelmed when I first spoke with her on the phone.

"We finally were given custody of our two grandchildren by the court last week," Peggy told me. "I think because their mother, my daughter Joan, was in jail on drug and child endangerment charges during the hearing. She agreed to sign over her rights. Harold and I were the only stable placement. We fought for our grandchildren so they wouldn't be placed in foster homes." She paused to catch her breath, or perhaps to cover the sound of her crying. I let her collect herself. "We want to do our best," she continued, "but I worry because the children have so many problems. We don't know what to do. We need help!"

I suggested she and Harold come in together for an intake appointment.

* * *

Peggy greeted me with a warm smile when I came into the waiting room. She was a rather large woman with a round face and short, cropped brown hair. Harold, a thin, older-looking gentleman with thick dark eyeglasses, sat next to her. Peggy politely introduced herself and Harold, and she said, "Thank you so much for seeing us today."

I asked them to come into my office. Peggy came in carrying a large binder, which she placed on the couch between her and Harold.

I said, "You told me over the phone you wanted both of your grandchildren seen for therapy."

Squeezing Harold's hand, she stated, "We realized we have been so focused on getting full legal rights to our grandchildren that we haven't gotten them the help they need. Javon has trouble controlling himself. Even though each of them has a bedroom, Javon sleeps with us. Jasmine has been crying, at times, for no reason."

Harold chimed in, "Our daughter Deborah told us over the weekend that we needed to get them help right away."

"Let me explain," Peggy said. "Deborah has them in her day care. She told us Javon acts like a feral animal at times. His behavior is unpredictable; he sometimes lashes out at his peers, hitting and throwing things. He has had to be removed and placed in the quiet space and held to calm him down. And Jasmine—Deborah said she mostly stays by herself with a sad and unhappy look on her face. Deborah told us she believed the children have been traumatized from the time they lived with their mother."

Peggy, a young grandmother in her early fifties, worked part time as a receptionist and now had become a mother again to two young children. Harold was a devoted husband who was still employed in the company he had worked at since high school. I said, "I can tell you both care very much for your grandchildren and want to do the best for them."

"My oldest daughter died in a car accident in high school," Peggy said. "Joan, the children's mother, is my middle child—she is a drug addict. My husband, Chuck, died of a heart attack when the children were young. He was a severe and chronic alcoholic until his death." Her face showed the strain of the many losses she had suffered.

Harold added, "We met after Chuck died. Deborah, our child together, is a day care provider. She has a stable marriage and has been helpful to us with our grandchildren."

I asked, "How much information do you have about Jasmine's and Javon's early history?"

Peggy picked up the three-ring binder and placed it on her lap. "I have everything here in this book. I have arranged the court papers and reports describing the children's early experiences in order. I feel more comfortable reading the material." She opened the book.

I noticed Peggy had highlighted sentences on the page. She started to tear up as she read out loud the results of the well-child checkup done at Joan's apartment: "Javon had marks on his chest. Jasmine crouched next to him as if trying to protect him. Both children appeared malnourished. The apartment was infested with fleas and bed bugs. Cats were all over the place. Javon sat in a dirty diaper. He had flea bites and some kind of rash on his legs. The police accompanied the social worker for this mandated unannounced visit."

I asked Peggy, "Do you have an idea when that report was made? How old were the children when the well-child checkup was done?" I knew such visits usually occurred when there were concerns of suspected child abuse and neglect. I wanted to establish a time line and understand the children's ages when the checkup was made.

"This report was written when Javon was a little over two years old." She turned to the next page and read: "Javon had tested positive for opioids and remained in the hospital for more than a week. There were ongoing concerns over the past couple of years about child neglect, continued failure to make the children's medical appointments, and a belief that the apartment was being used as a place for drug sales. A well-child check had been recommended."

I stated, "Joan probably didn't follow through on any of the report's recommendations."

"Of course not!" Peggy said. Her voice rose in pitch as she said, "I called Child Protective Services many times. I called the police. She refused to let us see our grandchildren. I was frustrated. I was unable to contact her. Her phone didn't work or she had changed her number as she usually did."

Harold sighed and said, "I still can't believe we went through all of this."

Peggy appeared distraught, as she too reflected on their ordeal. "Joan was a drugged-out mess. I know she was addicted to heroin. Her apartment was a haven for sick addicts. A disgusting way to bring up my grandchildren. I wanted to take the children to their doctor's appointments. I think she knew we had contacted the authorities. I think that was why she avoided us."

"About how long did this go on before the children were taken from their mother?" I asked.

She slowly and carefully turned the pages in the binder. This helped her gain some composure. She said, "I want to read from the report where the children were finally removed from their mother's care." She then stopped at a page and started reading: "The court filings concluded abuse and neglect. Both children were uncared for and showed clear signs of physical harm. When a social worker, accompanied by the police, entered the apartment, the mother and two males were passed out on the couch. The adults were unresponsive. The two children had been left unattended. They were subsequently removed from the household."

I asked, "How old were they when this happened?"

"Jasmine was five and Javon was three and a half," she said. Peggy again turned some pages in her book. I began to see not only that the binder contained significant early details about her grandchildren but also that having this difficult and overwhelming material organized together in one place was a comfort to Peggy. Reading the information allowed her enough distance from the facts so that she wasn't as emotionally triggered by her grandchildren's horrible early experiences.

She read more: "The children were residing in a neglectful and abusive environment. They were not safe and properly cared for. Jasmine would not make eye contact. She seemed to be caretaking her younger brother. She may have been physically and possibly sexually abused. The apartment was known as a drug den. Known predators and addicts inhabited the place."

When she finished, she looked up. "After being removed from their mother's, the children were placed with us for about six months during the court proceedings," she said. "Since no paternity was able to be established, Joan agreed to us obtaining legal and physical custody. Joan has to complete her jail time and a drug treatment program before she can even begin to have supervised contact with the children."

I talked to Peggy and Harold about the experience of trauma. I spelled out how early frightening events can have a severe impact on a child throughout their life. I said, "From the excerpts of the reports you just read to me, I can see your grandchildren were neglected and not cared for. They were left alone while the adults used drugs. I can't imagine what these little children had witnessed. They were brought up in an unsafe environment." I commended their attempt to provide their grandchildren with a safe and supportive home, and I explained to them that the best treatment would be to help the children feel as safe as possible and gradually learn to deal with the pattern of behaviors caused by the trauma they experienced.

"We love our grandchildren," Peggy said. "Since they have been with us, we have already seen some changes. They now enjoy being hugged. They wouldn't let us touch them when they first came six months ago."

We set up a treatment plan in which Ruth and I would provide a team approach. We had been in practice together for many years and would typically see siblings together when both children needed therapy. This made it easier on caregivers because they wouldn't have two different appointments in a week. We decided that Ruth would see Jasmine while I would see Javon. Peggy and Harold would participate in some of the children's meetings, and sometimes we would all meet together in one office for a family session.

* * *

At the next appointment, Peggy brought Jasmine and Javon for the children's first scheduled session. Ruth and I came out to the waiting room together, and I introduced Ruth to Peggy. I smiled at Peggy and the two children and asked her, "Who do we have here?"

Peggy said, "These are my grandchildren; this is Jasmine, and this is Javon." Jasmine sat very close to her on one side, while Javon clasped onto her arm on the other.

Javon was a sweet-looking interracial child, somewhat overweight for his short stature. His wide brown eyes had a look of dread when he saw me. He securely held his grandmother's hand. Jasmine was a thin, pale child with long, dirty-blonde hair and green eyes. She was a pretty little girl, but sadness seemed to radiate from her. Ruth said to her, "Jasmine, would you like to see what I have to play with in my office?" She was somewhat reluctant to go until Peggy reassured her, "You go with Ruth, I will be here; I won't leave you." She went with Ruth into her office.

I asked, "Javon, would you like to see all the toys I have in my office?"

Javon remained attached to his grandmother as the two of them followed me into my office. I said to Peggy, "I think Javon will like to play with some of my toys. Wait until he sees what I have to play with." They sat on my couch together, and he stared at the toys in the room.

Peggy started sharing her concerns. "Javon won't sleep in his own room," she said. "When I first got him he was skinny. Now he is always hungry. He eats everything in sight. You can see he's well fed."

As his grandmother told his story, I noticed Javon begin to show an interest in the toys. I gently walked over to the mutipurpose play table. I had taken the cover off because I had been doing sand play. I placed some cars and trucks in the sand. I asked, "Javon, would you like to come over and play?" He left his grandmother's side and sat on the small bench by the table. I sat next to him, and together we pushed the toy vehicles through the sand.

I said to Peggy, "Maybe Javon and I could play something together." Javon tucked his head in agreement as he moved a car through the sand. I asked

Peggy to give me some time alone with Javon, and I told her that she could come into the session later and tell me her concerns. She left my office while I had Javon engaged in play.

During his play, Javon made unusual noises, uttered guttural sounds, and displayed disorganized movements. He maneuvered the toy objects and banged the cars and trucks into each other. His manipulations were chaotic and nonimaginative.

I realized Javon never learned the positive benefits of play. Had the early trauma disturbed his ability to have fun? I had my first goal. I needed to help him experience the joy of play.

As he watched and intently observed, I demonstrated the rhythmic movement of the cars accompanied by driving sounds and noises. He seemed to relax. He then imitated my movements with sound. He repeated, "Vroom, vroom, vroom, vroom!" Carefully, he pretended to drive the vehicle around the sand without the crashes.

We engaged in the mindful calmness of movement as we drove our toy cars around the sand. We made up our own play rules. We waved to each other and smiled as we met during our travels. He said, "Hi!" He loosened up. We laughed together. He had some fun.

Abruptly, he stopped and pointed to something and called out, "What's that?"

I knelt down next to him and followed with my eyes the line of his little chubby finger, which beamed at the dream catcher hanging on the wall. I said to him it catches dreams. It's from a Native American reservation.

"What's it for?" he asked.

I explained that Native Americans believed it would help you sleep by catching bad dreams and letting the dreams go in the morning. He became absorbed by the object.

His eyes welled up, and he said, "Can it catch monsters?"

I asked, "Javon, do you have dreams about monsters?" Could this be why he wouldn't sleep by himself?

He said, "At night—when I sleep."

"What do they look like?" I was hoping he could tell me more so we could address some of his fears.

"They have big teeth!" he said.

We talked more about his nightmares. He said he felt safe from the night demons when he was sleeping with Mamie, as he referred to his grandmother. He said, "The monsters hide under my bed in my room." I said we can tell Mamie about the monsters and the dream catcher when we all meet. I connected with Ruth by phone, and she said they were ready to come into my office for the family meeting.

I opened the door to my office. Peggy sat in the middle of the couch, and just as they had done in the waiting room, the two children squeezed themselves close to her on either side. Javon grasped onto her right arm. Ruth took the chair next to the couch.

I started the family interaction by bringing up Javon's nightmares about monsters. "Javon said there are monsters with big teeth under his bed in his room," I said. "Peggy, maybe that's why he feels safer sleeping in your bed."

Peggy said, "I told him there are no such things as monsters; they are dreams, and they are not real."

I said, "It's important to help Javon feel safe." I suggested to Peggy that she put his mattress from his own bed on her bedroom floor to start with and then after a while she can move it into his room on the floor. "When Javon comes into your bedroom have him sleep on his own bed. There can't be monsters under the bed if it's on the floor," I said. His grandmother got it. She said she would get rid of the bed frame. She liked the plan to eventually have him sleep in his own room.

I pointed to the dream catcher hanging on my wall. "Javon would really like to have a dream catcher. He liked that they helped catch nightmares."

Peggy smiled at Javon and said, "I know where to get one of those. I'll get one for Jasmine as well. She's just getting used to being in her own room, but sometimes she ends up in my bed."

Javon looked pleased. Jasmine said, "Can we get one today?"

Peggy said to her, "We'll go later."

Ruth said, "Jasmine spent most of her time talking, playing, and worrying about Javon. My goal would be to help Jasmine learn to care more about herself." She turned to Jasmine and asked, "Did you like playing in my office?"

"I like coming here," Jasmine said. She turned to her grandmother and said, "When can we come again?"

* * *

Peggy brought the children regularly to their weekly appointments. Harold attended some of the appointments. The grandparents adapted to our treatment strategy. They became used to having separate meetings with Jasmine and Ruth in her office and Javon and me in my office. At times, we would have a family intervention with everyone present. Peggy was especially helpful in providing feedback and reflections on the children's behavior.

Javon's therapy during this time involved him learning to let go of the disturbing sounds, images, and noises of his past through play. Gradually, he enjoyed the freedom of fun activity without feeling restricted or worrying about his safety. The toy cars and trucks became his favorite expressive medium. We set up a repair shop and fixed broken cars. We shared and traded toy vehicles and developed a farm scene with the barn, cows, and horses. He occasionally had a startle reaction to a loud noise or an abrupt movement on my part or to something that just caught his eye.

One time as we were putting together the farm, he stopped, pointed, and, in a high-pitched tone, asked, "What's that? Is that a gun?"

I followed the projection of his finger to a toy *S*-shaped train track near the window. I went over and picked it up. I allowed him to touch the item. "Choo-choo-choo-choo," I said, mimicking the sound of a train.

He responded, "Choo-choo-choo."

I attempted to assure him that this was a safe place. "We have no guns here," I said to him.

In other sessions, Javon was able to relax from the interactive and positive rhythm of play. By learning to express himself through this medium, he could compensate for his shyness and inhibitions.

In one of our appointments, I took out a T. rex dinosaur with long teeth from the container of dinosaurs I had placed on the floor by the sand table. I said, "Let's pretend that this is the monster that bothers you at night."

He contemplated the T. rex for a moment and then grabbed four plastic stegosaurus figures from the container. He said, "We can get him with these."

I placed the T. rex in the sand, and he surrounded it with his figures. His figures jumped on my figure and defeated the T. rex by getting on top of him. I wondered about his nightmares. I asked him, "Are you still bothered by monsters?"

He puffed up his chest and said, "Monsters . . . don't scare me anymore. I'm not afraid of them."

* * *

After about a year of treatment, Javon had only an occasional nightmare. His grandmother reported that he was sleeping better at night and remained in his own bed in her room. Before long, he was ready to sleep in his own room. He had conquered his sleep issues. By that time, he was in first grade. It was at this time that Peggy brought up another concerning behavior.

She said in our family meeting, "I think he has an addiction to sugar, or sweets. He was caught stealing candy at my daughter's day care; he goes there after school. I found candy hidden under his bed."

We addressed the concept of addiction in families. We talked about how children who have addictive parents can have a vulnerability to addictive patterns of behavior such as intense cravings. We worked out a plan to counter his sugar cravings. She would allow him to occasionally have some candy. She would offer other choices for rewards and try to gradually fade out sugar.

Jasmine continued to make progress learning to focus less on her younger brother and more on herself. Peggy enrolled her in the third-grade soccer program, and Ruth soon reported that Jasmine seemed more confident.

"At first she told me she would worry about everyone else's positions," Ruth said at one of the family sessions. "She wanted to support her teammates. Through the insistence of her coach, she learned that securing her area was the best way for her to help the team."

Peggy confirmed that Jasmine appeared satisfied with her newfound interest in playing soccer. However, in the fall, when the soccer season had ended, Peggy came into a family session bewildered. Jasmine's teacher told her she had fallen asleep in class. At the same time, Javon's teacher was worried because he was caught stealing other students' snacks in the lunch room.

Why the change in both children's behavior? These were old behaviors that had been disappearing. In reviewing our notes, we established that this was around the same time of year the children were taken away from their mother. Peggy and Harold began to make a connection between the changes in Jasmine and Javon's behavior and other significant family events such as holidays and birthdays. Around these family celebrations, Jasmine would complain about difficulties sleeping, and she would end up being sad, tired, and irritable. Javon would crave sweets and would say insulting and nasty statements to Peggy and Jasmine.

Peggy labeled Jasmine and Javon's pattern of behavior their "trauma mode." The anniversary of a traumatic event had brought these behaviors out.

* * *

I was concerned about Javon's trauma reactions, and especially his intense arousal level. I introduced the breathing ball. This is a geodesic dome–shaped ball that can be folded and unfolded to help mimic the mindful movements of breathing. He learned to use it to calm himself in our session. I discussed beta-blockers with his grandmother. I explained to her that this type of medication was used for lowering blood pressure, and it could be helpful by lowering Javon's physiological arousal level during stress.

Peggy had been witnessing Javon's intense aroused level at home. "I ask him to come to dinner, and he flies off the handle! It's because of what he had to deal with as an infant. It's part of that trauma mode." She agreed to contact his primary care physician, whom I knew was understanding about providing medication to traumatized children.

After about a month on the medication, I observed Javon to have much better self-control. His play was more interactive, and he didn't become as easily frustrated when something didn't go his way. I asked him, "Are you able to come to dinner without yelling at your grandmother?"

"I don't do that anymore," he said. "Right, Mamie?"

Peggy said, "We haven't had a screaming incident in a number of weeks. I think something is working. He is even listening better. He doesn't get mad when I ask him to do something."

* * *

Jasmine didn't seem to have as serious of an anniversary reaction to being removed from her mother until she was in fifth grade. After the soccer season ended that year, she became grumpy and negative. On top of that, she wasn't sleeping well. She appeared to be stuck. Ruth worked with her on tapping, a form of therapy similar to acupressure in which she learned to tap on certain points on her body to relieve her stress. And she consulted with her primary care physician to place Jasmine on medication to help her sleep. When her sleeping improved, she was able to feel more positive and hopeful.

Ruth commended Jasmine in a family meeting: "Your negativity has shifted. I noticed that when you reflect on the past week's events, you don't always focus on the terrible things that happened. You seem happier."

Peggy agreed but still worried about Jasmine's negative attitude. "I think it's that trauma mode. When she comes home from school, she complains about the other students and the nasty teachers. Her life seems all bad."

Ruth offered a different parenting approach to Peggy. "What if you encouraged Jasmine to talk more about what good events occurred during school? Did she have a nice conversation with one of her friends? Did she learn something new? What did she have for lunch? Who did she sit with? Ask her if she could describe something good that happened."

"I can at least try," Peggy said. "I don't like when she comes home grumpy." She turned to Jasmine. "What do you think?"

Jasmine had been listening and said, "I know. I have to try harder and not worry so much. I worry that maybe I forgot to do some classwork or maybe the kids don't like me. I have to learn to accept that I'm okay. That's what Ruth keeps telling me to do."

* * *

Peggy and Harold maintained their commitment to raising their grandchildren. They worked on the parenting approaches we recommended, and throughout the years, the children consistently attended their appointments. The grandparents provided a positive and stable home, and Javon and Jasmine felt safe.

When Javon had just started middle school and Jasmine entered the ninth grade, a new concern emerged. Joan told Peggy the court deemed her fit to see the children. We were unsure if the children were ready for this. They had had limited contact with her and had shown no interest in talking to her when she would occasionally call during her incarceration.

The children were older. Jasmine had cut her hair short. She was muscular, while Javon was taller and chunky. After almost ten years, they were capable of making their own decision about seeing their mother in person.

Peggy laid out the situation in a family session: "Your mother has petitioned family court requesting to see both of you. Since Harold and I have legal guardianship and full legal rights over the two of you, it is our decision whether to allow her to see you. Of course, it would be up to what the two you wanted."

She went on to explain that their mother resided in an apartment that was watched over by the correctional department. She had no stable employment, but she had completed her drug treatment program and her jail time and was on parole.

"The visits would be supervised," Peggy explained. "Your mother's parole officer told me that an agency would monitor the visits. She said we could stop them at any time if they were harmful."

"Why now?" Jasmine said. "What if I don't want to see her?" She fidgeted with the hem of her sweater.

Her grandmother responded, "You have a point! She was allowed phone contact and could write letters during her time in jail. She would occasionally call, and she wrote me a letter asking for money a couple of years ago. She never asked about you or Javon until now."

We discussed the pros and cons of seeing their mother. The children were resistant to the visits, but they agreed to at least try a couple of supervised meetings. Since they hadn't seen her for a long time, I think they wanted to at least take a look at their mother. They wanted to see for themselves how she appeared.

"I guess I want to see Joan. To see if she is okay. I have nothing to say to her, though," Javon said.

"If he goes I will go, too," Jasmine said.

They both referred to their mother as Joan, possibly as a way of further distancing themselves from her.

Peggy consented to bring Jasmine and Javon to a space at the state office building set aside for monitoring and supervising family visits. She was not ready to see Joan herself. A supervisor would meet the children there so Peggy could avoid seeing her daughter. We planned a session after the interaction to debrief the experience. The family session went as follows.

Javon spoke first: "I don't think she knows how to be a mother. She didn't even ask me about school or anything. She didn't even know what grade I was in. She did show me her cell phone and told me her number. She said I should call her."

"I'm done," Jasmine said. "I don't think I want to see her again. She's nothing to me."

Harold said, "Things haven't been going well since the visit."

Peggy reflected on the past couple of days and said, "They haven't seen her in years. I thought seeing her would help, but it made things worse. It has been very difficult. I'm still picking up the pieces. Jasmine went to her room after the visit and refused to come down for dinner. Javon got in trouble the next day for mouthing off to his teachers."

In the end, the children agreed to try one more visit. I believe Javon was hoping things would be better. Jasmine felt she should accompany Javon.

But their mother missed this visit, and then she canceled the one scheduled after that.

In our next family session, Jasmine offered her view of what had happened. "On Facebook I found out Joan moved into an apartment with a new drug boyfriend. Her comments and posts on the page were all about alcohol and drugs."

Finally another supervised meeting was scheduled. Jasmine said she would attend this one because she didn't want Javon to go alone. In family treatment afterward, he said, "She wouldn't talk. She looked like she was falling asleep. Maybe she was on drugs. I think we should stop seeing her. She's just Joan to me. She's not a mother to me."

At this point, Peggy made an announcement. "That visit will be the last," she said. Joan's parole officer had let her know that Joan relapsed and had been charged with burglary, possession of stolen goods, and drug-related offenses. She was in jail again, and the visits with the children were suspended.

Peggy dabbed her eyes with a tissue and said, "I don't think she will ever get better. I feel sad that drugs are more important to her than her children. I'm thankful that I can be here for the two of you." Harold agreed.

Jasmine and Javon nodded in consensus to their grandmother's sad conclusion. Both appeared relieved not to have to see their mother anymore. Seeing their mother again, however, triggered Javon and Jasmine to want to process and explore the early life they had with their mother.

* * *

Within in our practice space, we have a small kitchen area and a café table with two chairs. This is where Ruth and I eat our lunch or take a break after sessions. It is also the place we use to process cases together. We felt we were at a transition point in Jasmine's and Javon's treatment and wanted to discuss our next strategy. We were sitting at the table having a cup of tea.

I said, "Javon is aware that his grandmother had a binder that had documents about their early history with their mother."

Ruth said, "Jasmine knows about it, too."

"Maybe, if Peggy consents, we could present the kids with the findings in the trauma binder," I suggested. "Having the information in a book has helped Peggy let go and detach from the traumatic memories. It could help them, too."

Ruth and I discussed the therapeutic benefits of reviewing the children's early events. Jasmine had early memories that Ruth was helping her cope with by using tapping techniques. She explained that about a year ago Jasmine brought up a frightening memory of a large man with awful, crooked teeth trying to touch her. She said that whenever she had this memory she became sad and afraid. When Jasmine told her about it, Ruth had Jasmine follow Ruth's fingers with her eyes as a way of calming her.

"She reported that the image was not as intense after I had used this procedure," Ruth said. "However, she was resistant to try it again. I believe it helped her because she never talked about that scary thought in the sessions that followed. I did get her to agree to use a safe therapeutic touch spot between her thumb and index finger when she needed to calm herself. I think she liked using pressure points better."

I shared that Javon had treatment resistance, too. He would use the breathing ball when he was younger, but after a while, he refused to use it. I taught him some deep-breathing techniques, but he said he didn't need them. He said he didn't need the medication anymore when he started middle school. Peggy agreed, and we decided to see how he would do without it. He appeared much better able to calm himself whenever he would become upset in our sessions. I asked how he calmed himself without using the medication. He took four deep breaths and told me this is the method he had figured out on his own.

"I believe there is often some treatment resistance that traumatized children have. It's like they become comfortable in their trauma mode!" Ruth said.

I agree, but added, "Still, learning to let go of their early trauma by hearing about it in an organized, contained package might help them define the experience. Then their emotions won't be stirred up by the trauma triggers, and their behavior won't be so focused on avoiding these feelings."

Ultimately, we agreed that Jasmine and Javon had progressed enough in their treatment to handle the material in the binder their grandmother had put together. They both had therapeutic tools to manage intense memories. We decided it would be best to present the historical data in the context of a family session.

Still sitting at our café table, we had finished our tea. We strategized how to best make it safe for Jasmine and Javon to hear about the history of their short life in their mother's care. Ruth planned to sit next to Jasmine to offer her support during the review of her early reported experiences. Any family member could immediately stop the conversation with a preplanned signal. We agreed on a raised flat hand movement. If necessary, we could take a break or stop the meeting or take calming breaths.

* * *

I previewed the family session concept with Peggy and asked her if I could borrow the binder for the meeting. She agreed to the plan and was appreciative that I was going to be the one reading the material and not herself. I went through the booklet and placed paper clips on the pages I was going to read from for the upcoming family session.

Finally, we discussed the idea of a family meeting with Jasmine and Javon. Jasmine, at this time, was discovering her potential as a high school athlete and excelled in several sports. But she was having trouble relating to some of her male classmates. As an attractive, athletic-looking girl, she felt that boys inappropriately invaded her space. She had shared with Ruth that boys made her feel uncomfortable. Javon, on the other hand, had found a nice peer group. He was a sensitive boy with a big smile. Both of them were ready to learn more about their early life with Joan.

We held the meeting in my office. I opened the door, and Javon, a broad-shouldered boy, entered first. I motioned to him to sit in the chair right next to the door. Jasmine saw Ruth smiling in a chair next to the couch, and she took a seat at the end of the couch closest to her. Peggy sat between the two kids, and Harold, the thinnest and slightest member of the family, sat at the end opposite Jasmine.

I sat in my office chair and opened the binder on my lap. Everyone stared at me with quiet anticipation. I prefaced the session by reviewing the safety plans that Ruth and I had established with Jasmine and Javon. I reminded them that the documents contained graphic details. The descriptions were based on police reports and Child Protective Services well-child investigations. Smiling at Peggy, I said, "Your grandmother has done a wonderful job at putting together all this information." This appeared to ease the tension in the room, so I started reading.

"No toys or playthings were noticed. The children appeared malnourished. The space was unsafe. Debris, food scraps, and clothes were scattered over the floor. The apartment had a significant odor probably from the old diapers on the floor. The baby was left unattended, crying in a broken crib with a dirty diaper. Rashes and blotches were observed on the infant's body. The other child hovered in the same corner as the baby's crib, appearing afraid and avoiding eye contact. The assumed mother made no attempts to comfort the children. She appeared bleary eyed and sat on the couch unaware of our presence."

Peggy couldn't hold back her tears even though she knew these details.

After a moment, Jasmine said, "Just what I expected. She was too drugged out to care for us. What a place to raise kids."

"Drugs were more important to her than us," Javon said. "Things haven't changed."

Looking at Jasmine, Ruth said, "I think you and Javon can understand why Peggy and Harold worked so hard at obtaining full legal custody of you both."

I said, "Peggy and Harold, you have helped make a stable and safe family for Jasmine and Javon for almost ten years. I believe they both are appreciative of what you have done."

I turned the pages in the binder to another section I had marked with a paper clip. This report contained information about the apartment being raided by drug enforcement agents.

"A warrant was obtained to search the apartment," I read. "A male identified as Bato was reported to be seen entering and leaving the premises. He was a known drug dealer and sexual predator. He had recently been released from incarceration. He was on parole with conditions. If found, he would be in violation of his release."

As soon as Jasmine heard this, she raised her hand—the signal that she needed to leave. Ruth took her into her office. I suggested to the remaining group that we had covered enough. The grandparents agreed, and I asked them to allow me time to help Javon process what he learned. I handed Peggy the binder and thanked her for letting me use it for the session. She and Harold went back out to the waiting room.

Javon appeared stressed but confirmed that listening to the reports about his early life validated what he felt. He took four deep breaths and then another four deep breaths. He then summed up his feelings.

"I have made a commitment to myself," he said. "I'm not going to use drugs. I hope to have a family. When I do, I'm going to be there for my kids. I don't care if I ever see Joan again."

* * *

A week later, I was in our kitchen making tea and waiting for Ruth to finish her session with Jasmine. Javon had finished his session, and I was wondering how Jasmine was doing. How did Jasmine handle the memories that were brought up by the reports? Was she able to process her discomfort?

Ruth came in and said she had some time for tea. She made some for herself. She grabbed her favorite Paris brand and poured hot water over it in her usual cup. As we sat sipping the tea at our little café table, I asked, "How was Jasmine doing?"

She had told me before that Jasmine was triggered by the drug raid report and memories related to Bato. Ruth had her use the acupressure point between her ring finger and pinkie to calm herself. Now Ruth said, "Jasmine believed Bato was the man in the terrible memory she described. In today's session, she talked more about the incident and his inappropriate actions with her. I had Peggy come in with Jasmine, and we called in a report together to Child Protective Services."

Ruth said today's session was a shift for Jasmine. "She talked about her discomfort with males, especially adolescent boys who only want sex and no relationship. She told me her feelings about boys didn't include the special relationship she had with her brother."

Ruth added that Jasmine seemed to gain some more understanding of her early life with her mother. "Jasmine said that the scary image was her fear. She had always felt afraid of men and everyone. Maybe, she told me, that was because she never felt safe with Joan." Ruth believed that sharing the binder in the family session might have helped Jasmine put her early trauma in perspective.

This was the only time the binder was presented in a family session. Neither Jasmine nor Javon asked to hear any more about the historical data in their grandmother's binder. The recapitulation of the early trauma ended one phase of treatment. We transitioned into a process where Javon and Jasmine engaged more in individual therapy.

* * *

In high school, Javon began to let go of his trauma mode. He admired the fact that Jasmine had been accepted into a local college and would play on the soccer team. He had grown into a tall, hefty, well-built adolescent and was actively pursued by the football coach to join the team. But Javon, unlike his sister, struggled with the concept of sports; he disliked competition, contact sports, and the jock culture. He became upset when the varsity coach insisted he needed to play football. He reluctantly agreed to practice with the team.

Javon said to me, "Coach Paisley wants me because I'm black. He was like, most football players in the NFL are black. You could be one of the bigger black players on our team. The workouts would help you build muscles and get rid of the pudge. You could make the team and do well."

Javon told me he felt Coach Paisley was prejudiced. He didn't like the kind of pressure the coach was putting on him to be part of the team. His large, strong physical stature tended to hide his sensitive, caring, and nurturing qualities. Javon didn't want to play sports. He told me one of his favorite things to do was to help his Aunt Deborah in the day care center. He said he really enjoyed playing with children.

Javon said, "I have trouble with physical contact. Maybe it's an early fear from the abuse, I don't know. But I don't think playing sports is my thing. My sister's thing is playing sports. I feel like I went through too many mean and nasty games when I was a child. I want to help kids. Helping others and having no drugs in my family is what I think I need to feel better."

Javon had struggled with aggression throughout his life. He usually maintained an inhibited and nonassertive stance. Telling the "football boss" (as he referred to his coach) he was not going to play would be a major step for him. Initially he chose to avoid the situation.

He said to me, "I just won't show up. He can't make me play."

Eventually, we decided to use this situation as a challenge to help him work through his passive stance. We role-played the scene with me pretending to be the "football boss." Javon laughed at the theatrics. After we worked on it, he agreed to confront the man and inform him that he was not into football.

At a later session, Javon told me how it went. "I did it!" he said. "I told him! I'm done. I just said to myself I was going to tell him, and I did it. Didn't even think about it. Like you said, just do it! And I did it! I even said he was prejudiced. He didn't know what to say. I told him goodbye."

* * *

Ruth and I were sitting at our space in the office. We were taking time to enjoy our tea together. We began reflecting on Jasmine's and Javon's experience of trauma. It had been a couple of months after the end of our treatment with them. We recalled how we had watched them change from frightened little children whose early life with their mother placed a significant burden on them. We reminded ourselves how their grandparents provided a safe home for them to grow into confident adolescents.

I said that Javon's learning to be more assertive was a game changer for him. He went to his guidance counselor and switched into the childcare program. He secured a part-time job working at his aunt's day care. He admitted toward the end of our time together that for him to be up-front, assertive, and honest would continue to be a challenge for him. He had evolved into a more open and confident adolescent despite the horrible early experiences he went through in his childhood.

Ruth washed out her teacup and set it in the rack. As she dried her hands on a towel, she reflected on Jasmine's final session. "I will not forget what Jasmine said at that session. She said that she felt she had awakened from her trauma and was now ready to move on with her own life."

CHALLENGES AND REFLECTIONS

The challenge of this case was the need for ongoing treatment for children who were traumatized early in their lives. Their grandparents remained committed to getting them that help. Ruth and I were able to work with Jasmine and Javon from early childhood until late adolescence. We helped them deal with their trauma behavior throughout the span of their development.

Javon was a frightened and inhibited child. He developed into a confident and sensitive teenager. In early childhood, he had difficulties with transitions. His reaction was one of fear, intense arousal, and an avoidance of the situation. This was his trauma response. I had to teach this four-year-old child how to play. He didn't know how to relax and have fun. I had to teach him to enjoy the soothing benefits of childhood play.

I started play therapy with making sounds and moving the toys around in different patterns of motion. I used a back-and-forth rhythm across his right and left visual field. I did this to integrate eye movement techniques into the play. This helped him feel calmer. Javon became engaged at this primitive play level. As our treatment progressed, Peggy shared that Javon began playing by himself at home. This basic play intervention worked. In time, Javon learned to play interactively.

Jasmine's trauma response was to protect Javon. At age five and a half, she began treatment with Ruth. She was terribly worried about her brother.

She talked about what had happened to him. She shared nothing about herself. Ruth helped her discover herself in therapy. Ruth said that Jasmine, as
a teenager, realized she was fearful and mistrusted men. This was due to an
early sexual incident. Jasmine by late adolescence accepted her early trauma
experience. She embraced a different purpose for herself. She wanted to go
to college. Unlike her mother, she wanted a career.

A turning point in Jasmine's and Javon's treatment was when Ruth and I
set up a family session. They were ready to review their early trauma. We
shared with Jasmine and Javon some of the details in Peggy's trauma binder.
The adolescents heard about the documented events they experienced with
their mother. They listened. They understood the impact of the terrible conditions they endured. After this family session, Ruth and I shifted our work
with them. We began seeing them alone as adolescents. The trauma binder
helped them gain a perspective of their early life. We refocused our treatment
to examine the meaning of their present experiences while being mindful of
their past.

Jasmine and Javon declared in treatment as teenagers that they were done
dealing with their mother. They didn't want to see her anymore. They needed
to detach from her. Javon made the decision that he was not going to repeat
her pattern of addiction. He wanted to be a better parent. Javon had become
more assertive. He confronted his football coach for being prejudiced.

Jasmine went through her own changes. She understood that her early
trauma experience would always be with her. She learned physical and behavioral coping strategies. Ruth believed that Jasmine was able to put her early
trauma in its place—like her grandmother did with the trauma binder. Jasmine
realized she wanted a different life than her mother had.

Peggy and Harold were devoted grandparents. Their challenge was to have
the hope that Jasmine and Javon would get better. Ruth and I offered them
as much support as possible. We helped them understand the dynamics of
developmental trauma. As co-therapists, Ruth and I supported each other. We
regularly processed our treatment and talked about our worries and successes.

Chapter 5

The Dollhouse

PRESENTING PROBLEMS

Jenny was a twenty-three-year-old young adult who decided she needed therapy. She stated she was having issues with trust in her relationships. She blamed her problems on her adoption and being raised by a lesbian couple. As her treatment progressed, she reexamined her early adoption memories. Jenny was adopted from a dysfunctional home. She was placed in a caring and nurturing environment.

When she began therapy, she was frustrated that her personal relationships were not healthy. As a child, she imagined her relationships would be like the figures in her dollhouse. In therapy, she learned as a young adult that her play fantasies were just the beginning of what she had hoped for. She realized that she had to work on forming caring and healthy relationships. These types of relationships don't happen on their own.

TREATMENT STORY

Jenny seemed anxious the first time she came into my office; she cautiously scanned the room with her large, brown eyes. She was dressed in dark slacks and a white blouse—professional attire—so I asked her if she'd come directly from work. She answered in a speedy, nervous burst.

"Yes," she said. "I'm always busy. I feel like I never have time for myself. I never get my work done. I seem to be in the office later than anyone else. I like the color of my office. Although it's not my favorite color. I like the color of this office. I think I would like to paint my office. Maybe I could paint it blue. If they let me I might change the color. Maybe after a while I can pick out new furniture. I always look at office furniture."

To ease her apparent nervousness, I explained the structure for treatment. I told her that this was a confidential setting. I wanted to help her feel safe. I hoped she would become comfortable telling me how she felt about her work and her life. I said, "Therapy is for you to talk about your feelings, your relationships, your perceptions, and yourself."

"This isn't my first time in therapy," she said. "But it *is* my first time choosing to go. I had to go when I was a child. I don't remember much about that time."

Based on our phone conversation the previous week, I knew she was twenty-three with a business degree and was working at a local ski center as the manager for booking. She hadn't offered me a specific reason for wanting to come in, so I asked her: "Why are you looking for help at this time?"

She responded, "I think I need to work on my relationships. I sometimes feel so alone. I just broke up with Bruce after two years. I don't know if I will ever find someone. I had trouble getting close to him. It feels like the same thing over and over again. A guy falls in love with me, but I can't seem to feel the same. I am adopted, and I was wondering if being adopted has messed me up. My caregivers are women. Does having two mothers affect how I relate to men? I guess I'm trying to figure out why I can't deeply trust."

"Did you think you felt closeness with your adopted family?" I asked.

"I was adopted after my sixth birthday by Tina and Miriam," Jenny said. "We celebrate the adoption date every year. This was the first year I couldn't go because I had to work. I think I had to go to therapy as part of the adoption."

"Do you remember much about your early experience of child therapy?" I asked.

She said, "It was a mandate by the state adoption agency. I recall being told I had an attachment problem. Tina and Miriam had to bring me. It was some kind of holding stuff, and they had to be part of it."

I wondered what sort of holding therapy she engaged in. Did she feel it helped her? I knew it was a long time in the past, but her reflections would allow me to understand more about her early relationships. I encouraged her to tell me more about this first therapy experience.

She confessed, "I didn't like the therapy. We had to hold each other. It made me feel uncomfortable. I had to put my arms around Tina and then Miriam. I remember it felt so artificial."

"Do you think this type of attachment therapy helped you in any way?" I asked.

She responded, "No! But it helped me gain respect for Tina and Miriam. I told them I hated going to the fake holding. They told me they didn't like going, either. Tina somehow managed to end the treatment. This really helped me accept them more as my parents. They listened to me."

I said to her that the memory she shared was ironic. "The fact that you stopped the holding therapy that was supposed to help you was what actually made you feel better." I laughed with her. I explained to her that that type of intervention is not supported by the research. Attachment problems in early childhood involve inadequate relationships with your primary caregivers, and holding each other is not going to make a difference in how you interact.

"However, your relationship with your caregivers actually did improve because they were responsive and nurturant," I said. "Tina and Miriam advocated for you to stop something that made you and them feel uncomfortable."

Jenny talked more about Tina and Miriam. "Miriam told me that a friend of my mother's cared for me as an infant. Apparently, my mother left before I turned two. She was an addict. Then I was placed in a couple of nonadoptive homes before I went to live with Miriam and Tina. They have continued to be supportive and helpful throughout my life. Miriam was extremely understanding when I asked her if I could change my first and last names when I turned sixteen. She let Tina know. It was Tina who assisted me through the legal stuff so I could change my name. My last name is a combination of their last names."

"So you are saying that you have developed a good relationship with your adoptive parents," I said.

She said, "Yes! I believe so. Tina and Miriam were more than caring. They understood my needs. They helped me when I struggled during adolescence to search for my biological parents. What was my mother like? Had she changed? I wanted to know. Miriam was so comforting. I was sad and hurt. In the end, it was Tina who was able to locate my mother. She discovered she was a prostitute and still an addict. I was just in shock. I couldn't believe it! I decided I didn't want to see her. My biological father could never be clearly identified. I was done with them. Tina and Miriam were my parents."

I thanked her for sharing her memories. I asked if she recalled anything more about the early years of her adoption. I was curious to learn what other thoughts she had regarding the experience.

She seemed to be staring at something in the corner of my office. "I still have a dollhouse like that," she said. "I would play family with it when I was little. I was given the gift of family. Miriam and Tina wanted to be a family and have a child to raise. I never felt like I had a home until I met them. I think we found each other."

Jenny appeared happy about her family life. I worried she thought that because she didn't have a biological connection to Tina and Miriam this would cause her to have poor attachments to people. I believed that she felt that being adopted affected her relationships. I asked, "Do you think that because Tina or Miriam aren't your biological parents that you won't be able to trust them?"

Her large brown eyes welled up, and she disengaged from eye contact. "We had a big fight a couple of weeks ago because I couldn't get off from work to celebrate my adoption day. They seemed upset. I had this feeling that they didn't care for me. I was worried. I think it might have to do with something before I was adopted. All I wanted was a caring family."

I was thinking that we should continue to establish her adoption as a healthy process. I asked, "Do you have other good memories about your adoption?"

She appeared to give this some thought and said, "I always remember wanting to be adopted. I had all these different caregivers. I wished each one would have been my family. But it felt like no one wanted me. All I wanted was to have a real family. Then I was placed with Tina and Miriam. As soon as I moved in, I felt cared for. I wanted them and they wanted me."

"Your adoption was important," I said.

"You know, I never really shared the details of my adoption with Bruce," she said, "but I'm done with him."

We completed our first session. Jenny had managed to recall some memories about her adoption, and she had become comfortable sharing her feelings and reflecting on her relationships.

* * *

In her next session two weeks later, she was dressed more casually. She sat in the same chair she had before and crossed her legs at her ankles. "Today, I went home and changed from my work outfit," she said.

"You seem more relaxed. I think you helped me understand your adoption last time," I said.

"It wasn't easy," she said. "I had never talked about my adoption with anyone. Few of my college friends knew about Tina and Miriam."

"What was your childhood like after being adopted?" I asked.

"I grew up in this small town in northern Vermont. I see the few friends I went to school with when I go home to see my parents. Tina spent her life in the area. She is a supervisor in a local factory. Miriam does respite for the elderly. She met Tina in the big city of Burlington. Everyone knew about us, but nobody ever talked directly about us. I think we were accepted. Miriam and sometimes Tina would come to school events. The three of us were a family, and were part of our small community."

"It sounds like you felt the security of family with Tina and Miriam. What was your relationship with them like?" I asked.

Jenny conceptualized her relationship with Miriam by sharing the following image, "I think of my biological mother as a frozen snow woman. I never knew her. Miriam became the goddess of warmth that melted her."

I said, "You express such a nice feeling of warmth and nurturance when you talk about Miriam. What is Tina like?"

She said, "Tina is direct. She tells it like it is. When we would cuddle on the couch, I would lie on Miriam's lap. Tina had her own chair. But when anything needed to be done, Tina took care of it. I liked helping her with projects around the house. We painted the deck together."

"What is one of your fondest memories of your family being together?" I asked.

She said, "Our first Christmas together. They bought me a dollhouse. Like the one you have there. I remember playing for hours. I set up the furniture in the house. I recall arranging each room. I put the toy figures in the rooms. I would have the play people sit around the dinner table. I imagined that this must be what a real family was like."

Jenny was able to have a make-believe family in her dollhouse. She felt when she was a child that adoption would solve everything and help her have the family relationships she wanted. But it didn't make the rest of her life all better. She now had a career and was living on her own, but again she had that lonely and unhappy feeling after breaking up with Bruce.

"Why do you think you weren't able to get close to Bruce?" I asked.

"I think he became too controlling. He was a trainer at a gym where I went to college. In the beginning, he was great and helped me develop a workout routine. When I moved away for my job, we continued to see each other. He would text me every day and ask if I had trained. Then when he came to visit me he would like check me out to make sure I was working out. He was addicted to exercise. I didn't like it. It didn't feel like a good relationship, so I told him I was done."

She said, "I wasn't able to connect with him and never cared as deeply about him as he said he felt about me." She had blamed the adoption. She was ashamed about having two mothers and growing up in a small town.

* * *

Jenny wanted to work on the quality of the relationships she had now. In order to do this, I believed she had to change how she saw her adoption. Tina and Miriam were not doll figures; they were real people. They cared about her, and she cared about them. This is the true trust and security of family.

In this next phase of treatment, I worked with Jenny on the rhythm of reflecting on the positive memories and images she shared about her childhood when she felt lonely and abandoned by her friends. I helped her construct a feeling of safety about her adoption and her family. When she felt ungrounded and worried or thought none of her friends cared for her, I suggested she should balance herself by recalling these positive images. The problems and challenges in her current relationship persisted. She was worried that after her relationship with Bruce that she would never be able to get close to anyone.

* * *

In a follow-up session, Jenny came in wearing her business outfit. She sat up straight in her chair, gritting her teeth and seething. "Mr. Cross, my boss, didn't give me a raise," she said. "He gave Erik, my male coworker, one. I know because Erik told me so. I hate my boss. He's a narcissist like most men. They only care about themselves. I want to quit. I can't stand my job."

She was extremely agitated. I encouraged her to sit back and take some calming breaths. I talked about her safe memories and thinking about Miriam as the goddess of warmth. As she relaxed, I reminded her about her dollhouse, how Tina and Miriam weren't dolls and that she had to work on the relationship. When she had become more comfortable, we reexamined the current situation.

She said, "I thought I would get a raise. I believed I was doing a good job. When I didn't get it, I didn't know what to say. I guess I didn't say anything. Erik said I should talk to Mr. Cross, but I didn't think I could face him."

"I think this might be a relationship you could improve on," I suggested. "Maybe you could assert yourself with Mr. Cross and explain to him why you deserve a raise. Could you think of a way you could talk with him?"

She crossed her ankles again and sat back in the chair. She said, "I need to present the facts. I have the data to show him. I have increased bookings. I will give him the reasons I should get a raise. If I don't get one, I will quit."

"That's a much better approach!" I said. She committed to setting up a meeting with her boss. We role-played what she could say to him. I advised her not to quit her job until she had another one. She smiled at me and said, "I wouldn't do something like that."

* * *

Jenny canceled her next appointment and then canceled the one after that. I began to wonder if this was her way of not returning to therapy. Finally she made another appointment and came in wearing her business suit again. "What happened?" I asked.

She said, "I wanted to talk with Mr. Cross before I came in again. But it was hard to arrange a meeting with him. Finally I did it. It was a task I had to do. I clearly presented the facts and numbers to show the increase in bookings and my benefit to the company. Guess what? I ended up with more of a raise than I expected."

I noticed a change in her demeanor as she described her meeting with her boss. Usually when she had on her work clothes, she would sit up straight so as not to wrinkle the outfit. But this time she folded herself back in the chair with a pleased look on her face. "You asserted yourself with Mr. Cross, and it made a difference," I said. "You were direct and to the point. The way you were direct reminds me about what you said about Tina in her relationships."

"I have never felt confident around males that were in positions of authority," she said. "I thought about my interactions with some of the male college professors I had. I would only talk with them when I was well prepared and had my facts straight."

I raised the issue of her relationships. "It seems like you want to work on improving your interactions with men," I suggested.

She said, "I have always felt safer with women. Maybe because I have two female caregivers. I don't know. But I do know I am sexually attracted to men. I fantasize about relationships with them. I think I have to learn to trust men more."

I reminded her about her relationships with her caregivers. She felt safe in her family of choice, and even though she didn't have a biological connection, she learned from them. I said, "I'm guessing you must have learned how to be direct and assertive from Tina."

* * *

During the next several sessions, we focused more on Jenny's social relationships. I asked about her friends during her school years.

She recalled, "I had a stable peer group all through school. I'm still in contact with a few of my friends from high school. But you don't get to really know each other. It was like a comfort group, you know? You feel that in a small community. We did activities together, but we didn't share anything real."

Next, I attempted to understand more about her romantic interests. I asked questions about boyfriends and her sexual experiences.

"My boyfriend in high school took me to senior prom," she said. "Everyone went. He was my first sexual experience. It was safe because we only engaged in oral sex. The relationship ended when I went to college."

"What were your relationships like in college?" I asked.

She said, "In college, I took more chances. I experimented more. I partied. I tried to be less inhibited. But I was always on the watch. I was somewhat evasive with the guys I met. I think I only saw them for their looks. Like I didn't totally trust them. I was guarded. I had trouble allowing myself to enjoy the relationship."

"You talked before about your problem with trust. Can you tell me more about this feeling?" I asked.

She said, "I worry about getting close to people. I feel if I get close they will only leave me. I think it has to do with the image I had of feeling so alone before I was adopted. I felt I had no one. I had no family. No one cared for me. I felt all alone." She wiped her eyes as she sat back. I was about to get the box of tissues. She said, "I'm okay."

We processed these haunting and recurrent negative feelings she had about being alone before she was adopted. I wanted to give her a tool to deal with these feelings. I talked to her about some tapping techniques, other nonverbal strategies, and mindfulness mediation. She was intrigued by the idea of tapping.

I said, "Tapping focuses on meridians or energy centers in our body. By putting pressure or tapping on these areas, you can reduce the stress you feel from negative emotions."

"I've heard about pressure points you can press on to relieve stress," she said.

I demonstrated the twelve meridian points on each side of my body that correspond to an internal organ. We practiced the sequence of taps together. I had her focus on the alone feeling while accepting positive images of her adoption and the dollhouse. She went through the tapping sequence.

"How do you feel?" I asked afterward.

She said, "I don't have that terrible feeling of being so alone. It doesn't feel as intense."

She planned to use this technique when she needed to reduce the effects of her sad and intrusive feelings of aloneness.

* * *

Jenny continued to regularly attend her sessions. She worked hard at countering her worries about being alone. At one session after a year of treatment, I asked more about how she was managing her friendships. She said, "I think I'm dealing better with my close friends. I'm trying to stay present. When I start feeling insecure about someone, like if I worry that they don't like me or don't care, I take a breath and let it go."

Jenny's early feeling of loss and abandonment had had a strong impact on her. I believed it left her with a deep-seated feeling of mistrust in her relationships. I said, "That feeling of aloneness from your early life still affects your relationships."

Jenny, who usually maintained her composure, began to tear up. "Yes, I have this fear of being alone. I remember worrying that Tina and Miriam would send me away if I didn't listen. I have always worried that my friends would leave."

I offered her a tissue. "Are you getting better at handling those feelings?" She listened and wiped tears away. "Yes, I think so. It's been more than a year since I ended my relationship with Bruce. I feel I did the right thing by telling him I was done. I don't feel so alone. I like me. I feel I am a stronger person because of my adoption."

* * *

This change in Jenny's realization led to the next phase of treatment. She began to let go of her fear of being alone. We were able to focus more on her current social network. She was able to understand and uncover when her old pattern of loss and fear of abandonment affected her present interactions.

She said, "I think I have been getting better about moving on. If I worry someone doesn't like me anymore, I say to myself, "Here goes that old feeling again." I say goodbye to the loss feeling and let it go. I say to myself, "If they don't like me, so what. It's their loss."

In a later session, she seemed to have a setback. She leaned forward in the chair and began to lament, "I hate my job. I can't stand any of my coworkers. I need to move. My roommates are annoying. Nothing is going right. Why should I bother coming here?"

After her burst of negative energy, I encouraged her to reflect on her statements. "Is that your feeling of loss coming back to haunt you again?" I asked.

She said, "I came today prepared to talk about my friendships. But somehow I became overcome with sadness. I felt defeated. Like nothing was going to help."

We went through the tapping sequence she liked, and I encouraged her to let go of her disappointments. I said, "Let us put your life in perspective. Where are you in your development? You have secured a job in your career, you moved into your first apartment after college, and you have established a new social network. You have done very well for yourself."

She thought for a moment as she slouched back into her chair. "Yes, but I have to accept that relationships are a work in progress. I am trying to be more honest and open with my friends. I need to believe in what I have accomplished."

"What about your relationships? How are things going?"

She said, "I have been having lunch with Erik. We eat together almost every day. We seem to be able to talk about all sorts of things. I enjoy him. But he's not my type."

"What do you mean?" I asked.

"He's overly sensitive and nerdy," she said. "He does the graphics for the company. But he's ten years older than me. He's not built like Bruce. Bruce was into his muscles and was quite buff. The kind of man I am usually attracted to."

We were not having another session for several weeks. She was spending some time with Tina and Miriam. I wanted to leave her with something to contemplate before that next meeting. I proposed she think about taking social risks. I suggested she attempt to move out of her usual comfort zone. Don't let the worry of loss inhibit your relationships. Be honest and trust in yourself, I advised her.

* * *

Upon her return, I asked how the visit with her parents went.

"There were some good times and not-so-good times," she said.

"What do you want to tell me about first?" I asked.

"Well, it always happens," she complained as she sat straight up. "Miriam was so nurturing and pleased with what I've achieved. Then Tina tries to control everything. She tells me I can do better. Miriam was so supportive, but Tina makes me feel like I'm nothing. Why do I go home? I should just stay here. I should never see them."

I said to her that she was allowing her negative feelings to delude her thinking. Gradually her anxiety quieted down, and she became grounded. "How can you reframe your relationship with your parents?" I asked.

She reflected, "Miriam—I know she cares very much about me. Tina comes on harsh, but that's who she is. She is direct and to the point, and I know she means well."

"That's better," I said. "You need to see the positive and negative aspects of your parents' interactions. Some things about them you won't be able to change. But if you feel that Tina's bluntness affects you, tell her."

As she thought more about her family, she said, "I enjoyed the meals we had together. I had a feeling of comfort. I realize I can't change some things about my parents. But I have been trying to be more honest."

"What do you mean?" I asked.

She explained, "I did tell Tina that her directness sometimes is hurtful. I told her I thought she didn't care if I came home for my adoption day. She immediately responded. She said she was sorry. She told me she didn't know it upset me. She really wanted me to come home, but she said she had to accept that I couldn't leave work. She said she just tells it like it is. 'I am just a plain-speaking person,' she said."

"That was a candid and sincere conversation you had with Tina," I said.

"Her response restored my faith in being honest. I need to trust that my parents care about me. I need to be confident that if I tell them what bothers me they won't abandon me."

I saw that she was more relaxed and comfortable talking about herself than when we first met. I pointed out how when she first began treatment she would go into too much detail about events, and not talk about herself. I commented on the attractive eyeglasses she was now wearing, along with her colorful outfit. Did she feel differently? Did she notice a change in herself that I saw?

She said, "When I first started coming in, I felt upset and negative. I feel more centered and balanced now. Maybe when my relationship with my parents doesn't feel good, I feel out of whack as well. I miss them. I appreciate having them as parents."

I noticed Jenny intently staring at my dollhouse. I asked her what she was thinking.

"I'm thinking about my own dollhouse. When I was home, it was in my room. My parents saved it along with other items of my childhood. I still think about playing with that dollhouse. Putting the toy family together at the dinner table was what I dreamed of. This time when I went home, I knew what I always wanted was a loving family. But I also realized that the real relationships I have with Tina and Miriam are important, too."

I recognized that Jenny had discovered the meaning of her adoption story. She had put together that her lack of trust in her current friendships was affected by a feeling of loss and abandonment in her pre-adoptive years. This led her to engage in a pattern of keeping her friends at a safe distance to protect herself. I said to her that realizing she has trusting and supportive parents has helped her confidence. She wholeheartedly agreed.

She said, "I need to get out of my comfort zone socially. Maybe I should try something different."

* * *

She said to me in a later session, "Guess what? I'm dating Erik. I know I said he wasn't the kind of man I'm attracted to. He's thin and not very athletic. My God, he even wears casual clothes," she added with a self-deprecating laugh.

"What about the quality of the relationship?" I asked. "Can you trust him? Can you be honest with him?"

She said, "I'm enjoying our conversations. He's sensitive. He asks me how I am, and he seems like he sincerely wants to know. We can talk about our families. We talk about everything. I told him about my adoption. He comes from a stable family. I feel we have an honest and open interaction. I feel close to him."

She seemed to have a trusting relationship with a man. She even invited Erik to meet her parents. She told me that she worried that she would lose him once he met them. It was that old feeling. Would he not like her once he saw she had two mothers and realized she was adopted? Instead, they happened to really enjoy each other.

In our last meeting, Jenny admitted that the feeling of abandonment would still come to her at times. But she had learned to accept it. She did tell me she used her tapping to help her let the feelings go. I believed Jenny's adoption helped her develop a deeper understanding of relationships. The strength she gained from her relationships with Tina and Miriam helped her overcome the pattern of loss and abandonment she sustained in her early, pre-adoption years. I believed that, by continuing to work on her relationships, she would eventually be able to develop a real family for herself and leave her dollhouse to her children.

CHALLENGES AND REFLECTIONS

Jenny as an adopted child was placed in a loving and caring family with Tina and Miriam. She had feelings of loneliness and self-doubt from her early adoption. This remained a theme for her as a young adult. As a little girl, she found safety in her play. She played out the fantasy of a stable family in her dollhouse.

Jenny had a difficult first therapy experience as a child. My treatment challenge was to help her to feel safe in our therapeutic relationship. As she became comfortable, she shared her psychological story. She blamed her adoption and having two female caregivers for her problems. She learned that it was her own negative thoughts about these experiences that affected her social relationships. Jenny as a young adult realized that she had to make an effort to have healthy relationships.

Jenny made a commitment in her treatment to be honest and open in her relationships. She began this change by expressing her concerns to her parents. She talked to them about the quality of their family relationships. They listened and appreciated what she had to say. They began to understand each other.

This family encounter helped Jenny become confident about her perceptions and feelings. She realized that blaming others for her problems was not helpful. Jenny recognized that she had to be responsible for herself. The therapy helped her trust in herself.

Chapter 6

The Problem of Divorce

PRESENTING PROBLEMS

A divorce can affect parenting and a child's behavior. Having two house-holds means the children in this family received mixed messages about their actions. Nicole and Gary, the parents, competed with each other to see who was the better parent. They didn't share their perceptions or talk about their children with each other. The three children were parented by Nicole and Gary in an inconsistent manner.

In their treatment, eight-year-old Dominic, ten-year-old Bradley, and fifteen-year-old Mariah spelled out their problems being in a split family. This was explained to their parents. Mariah was a strong, independent teen-ager. She decided to confront Nicole in family therapy about the problem of living in two homes.

Nicole and Gary agreed to come in together for parenting advice. Ruth and I tried to help them understand their children's concerns. They listened to some helpful strategies. Nicole and Gary made parental changes. They adjusted the visitation schedule to accommodate the needs of their children.

As co-therapist in this case, I knew it was important for me to have an understanding of the effects a divorce can have on children. I saw Dominic and Bradley while Ruth saw Mariah in therapy. We engaged Nicole and Gary in the children's treatment. Ruth and I processed what happened in our treat-ment. Our goal was to help the parents understand the needs of their children and come up with common parenting strategies.

TREATMENT STORY

Nicole contacted our practice looking to set up therapy for her three children. She had recently divorced and wanted to get them help. I thought to myself, *Another divorce case.* I always feel concerned for the children in split families. They tend to blame themselves. The hurt and troubles surrounding divorce are not their fault.

I approached Nicole in the waiting room with the intake packet. Her thin, jittery, neat appearance was accompanied by the odor of cigarette smoke. I handed her forms for each of her three children, and she busily completed the paperwork. After she came into my office, I explained the process of child and family treatment.

I asked about her reason for requesting therapy for all her children. I wanted to begin to establish my role as an advocate for the children's best interests. I explained that I would need input from both parents. I made it clear that I wouldn't be on either parent's side. I said, "I will determine your children's needs and help you and your ex find the best way to co-parent them."

She thought about what I said. She sat straight up, managing to use only the small front edge of the chair. She announced, "My lawyer told me to get the children counseling. He told me my children may need help learning to deal with living in two homes."

I asked, "Where are you in the legal process?" I was hoping the case was settled; I would have some reservations about getting involved if it was still in court and undecided. I don't like to be drawn into testifying in divorce cases if I am providing treatment.

Nicole answered, "Finally the court stuff is over—our case is done, and we have an agreement. It all cost way too much! I am especially worried about Mariah, my oldest, she's fifteen, and Dominic, my eight-year-old. Bradley, who's ten, seems to be okay."

"What are your concerns?" I asked. I attempted to gather information from her perspective knowing that the father and even the children may see things differently. This is an impact of severed households. Due to the split relationships, everyone tends to see things from their own point of view. There is often a lack of sharing between families, and each parent tends to believe that they are the one with the better household.

"Mariah says that her father is always working, and Dominic says he is never around," Nicole said. "Bradley doesn't complain. None of the kids want to go to his house. They like hanging out more at my boyfriend Jimmy's trailer. We let them do what they want. Their father has too many rules."

These critiques didn't surprise me. In divorced families, children are always caught in the middle and sometimes feel they are the cause. They also want to please their parents. Therefore, a child may have a tendency to go along with one parent's criticisms of the other parent or voice complaints to make the parent happy. I asked Nicole about the custody arrangement.

At last she sat back in the chair and seemed to slightly relax, although she managed to spell out other concerns related to the children's father.

"Gary and I have joint custody. I told him I was coming here. He didn't say anything to that. I think he would agree to the children getting counseling. You never know with him."

I questioned her about the state of their postdivorce communication. This was important because her children could easily take advantage of their parenting rules if they don't talk with each other. I said, "Do you and Gary have conversations about the children and share common rules about bedtime and homework? This usually helps your children not take sides or split the two households up. It also helps set up more consistent rules for the children."

She almost jumped at me. "I don't talk to him! We still fight. We just can't get along. Whenever I try to talk to him, he yells. We pick the children up at school so we don't have to see each other. This way he can't yell at me."

I began to worry because she reported having conflictual interactions with the children's father. I believe that frequent conflicts between the parents increase the children's stress levels.

I inquired about the court-mandated visitation plan. She explained that it was a three-day four-day arrangement. "I get them for three days, then he gets them for four days, then I get them for four days, and it continues this way. This causes problems when the change comes over the weekend. We have to see each other. Then we start arguing."

I wondered if they were able to work through any postdivorce conflict. What is their problem-solving ability? I was concerned about the children witnessing their parents' arguments. I asked, "How do Gary and you handle the situation when you have to pick up the children at the other parent's household?"

She said, "We stay in our cars. That way we don't have to talk. The kids go into his place on their own. So far it has worked."

"What about medical appointments and school meetings? Who takes responsibility for them?" I asked. I was trying to understand her role and whether pertinent information about the children was shared.

She insisted, "I'm the one who takes the kids to the doctors. I deal with school. Gary doesn't take care of anything. I do it all. He never asks me about the doctor's visits or school."

She didn't identify any problems the children had other than the divorce. I wondered what effect the parents' conflicts had on the children. What did the children witness? How long had they experienced their parents' marital conflicts? I decided to ask a more pointed question: "When do you think your marital difficulties began?"

She scooted back onto the chair's rear seam, uncrossed her legs, made eye contact, and said, "We started fighting right after Dominic was born." Smirking slyly, she said, "He says the kid is not his. We won't know the truth, as he refused to have a blood test."

"So that's when you and Gary began to have conflicts?" I wanted to understand how unstable their relationship was.

"I was pregnant with Mariah during my senior year in high school. I had to drop out. I finished school in a program for pregnant teens. Gary and I decided to get married after she was born," she said. "Yeah, and guess what? It was all bad. All we did was fight and argue. I stayed home with the children. He worked at the flooring and tile store. He's the manager now. We didn't see much of each other. When we did, it was yelling and screaming. Nothing physical, or I would have called the police. He knew I would." She tensed her jaw and nodded, more to herself than to me.

"You managed to have two more children and stayed together," I said to her. I realized the children apparently experienced a conflict-filled relationship in their parents' marriage for fourteen years. That's a lot of chaos for children to deal with. "Why did you finally decide to get a divorce?"

"I couldn't take it anymore. He wasn't coming home. We couldn't talk to each other. I went to a lawyer. The divorce seemed to take forever. I moved into my mother's with the children about three years ago. It took two years to finally get an agreement," she said with a sigh of relief.

"What are the current circumstances of the children's households?" I asked.

"I've been working as a receptionist for an insurance company for the past couple of years," she said, smiling. "I live at my mother's house. She helps with the kids. My boyfriend, Jimmy, has two boys. James is eleven, and Evan is eight. We spend a lot of time at his trailer. The kids like going over there. They go four-wheeling in his woods."

"What about Gary's household?" I asked.

"Gary lives with his girlfriend, Kate. The kids say they don't like her. She doesn't have any children. She treats the kids like they're hers. They tell me she is mean. She makes them do their homework right after school and they can't play until it's finished. They say she spends more time with them than their father does," she complained.

I complimented her for presenting a picture of her children's family situations. Since the divorce resulted in a joint custody agreement with equal decision power, I informed her that both she and Gary would have to consent to the treatment. I explained that since three children were involved, Ruth and I would probably provide co-therapy. Nicole was comfortable with this approach. One of us would contact her with the next appointment.

*　*　*

After Ruth met with Gary, we compared the information we had gathered from our interviews with the parents. We wanted to review each parent's perceptions to develop an understanding of the family patterns. We processed the details before we had our appointments with the children.

Ruth explained Gary's take on the situation to me. "In regard to their relationship, Gary admitted he had trust issues with Nicole from the beginning of their relationship. He believed she cheated on him with Jimmy. He accepts Dominic as his child, regardless of paternity. He didn't need to get a blood test. He met Kate several years ago. He reports having a caring and supportive relationship with her. She wants to be a part of the children's upbringing. Kate is unable to have children."

We identified the parenting issues. Nicole appeared to be jealous of Gary's relationship. She didn't like that Kate was involved with her children. Nicole believed the children didn't like going over to their father's place. I expressed my concern that Nicole portrayed Gary as not a good father.

Ruth offered a differing viewpoint. "I believe Gary has a commitment to the children, but he has limited understanding of how to parent. He admitted to me in our session that his father was never involved with him. Therefore he said he never learned what it meant to be a father. He expressed some confusion about his oldest daughter to me. He told me that she complains about her mother being too controlling and bossy. And he said that Dominic doesn't like going over to Jimmy's trailer. He was worried because Dominic said Jimmy's boys pick on him and don't let him ride the four-wheelers."

We began to realize how their divorce had caused splits in the family relationships. Nicole and Gary didn't trust each other. They were hearing concerns from their children but weren't sharing the information with each other. They didn't know how to parent together. We hoped that, by advocating for the children's best interests, we would be able to help the parents empathize with their needs. Ruth would work with the oldest daughter. I would see the boys. We would involve the parents. We knew Gary and Nicole would not come in together. Our goal would be to improve communication between Nicole and Gary about the children to help establish a more consistent parenting approach.

*　*　*

Dominic came in for his first session with his mother. As I approached him in the waiting area, his mother offered some peculiar encouragement. She urged him, "Tell the doctor what's the matter. You can tell him your problems."

Dominic was a slight child. He seemed a little unsure about coming into my office. So I said, "I have toys in my office I want to show you, and you can play with." As he walked in, he was immediately attracted to the drawing board. Standing transfixed in front of the display, he scanned each picture.

His blue eyes widened as he recognized a picture and pointed to it and said, "That's a Ho-Oh." This is a rare avian-type Pokémon similar to a peacock with gold and red feathers not easily identified by most children. I was impressed that he knew the character. I gently asked him if he would like to sit at the children's table and draw. He responded with a nod and smile. I gathered the drawing materials and placed them in front of him. We talked about Pokémon.

He said, "I like Pokémon. I play Pokémon Sword and Shield the most. I capture all the different Pokémon." He carefully selected a piece of blank paper and started outlining a figure on it.

I maneuvered myself across from him into my chair at the play table. As he became calmly engrossed in drawing, his half smile endured while he maintained his focus on rendering his picture. I became interested in what he planned to draw.

He said slowly, "I'm—going to draw a Raichu. It is my favorite. It evolves from Pikachu. It stores electricity." He picked out orange-, brown-, and yellow-colored pencils.

As he worked on a picture of a rodent-like creature, I asked him about his two households. I wondered, "What is it like living in different houses?" He didn't respond. "Your parents don't live together?" He continued to draw. I believed he might have difficulty expressing himself with words. He finished his drawing, and I placed it on the board. He was quite pleased.

Since he liked drawing, I suggested he try to draw the different places where he slept. He seemed interested in putting something else on paper. I thought that with his strong visual processing ability maybe he could better represent his concerns.

He said, "Three places; I sleep at my dad's, my grandmother's, and the trailer."

I placed three sheets of blank paper on the table. "Which place would you like to draw first?" I asked.

He stated, "I will do Dad's place." He began to outline his father's home. As he started to sketch the interior, I asked if he could identify who slept in each room. He placed his sister in her own room. His brother and he were adequately drawn sticklike figures placed next to each other in a shared space. The siblings were all drawn as residing in the upstairs portion of his rendition.

He sketched a large square and stated, "This is my dad and Kate's room. It's a big room downstairs."

He penciled in a small yellow cat and a brown dog in his and his brother's room. He continued to demonstrate a knack for visual expression. I thought that maybe I could get him to talk through his pictures. I asked him about his father's home. I placed my finger on the picture. "What do you like most about your father's place?"

He said, "My room at Dad's is my best space." I asked him which sleeping place he would like to draw next. He said, "Grandmother's!"

He methodically made a large square for his grandmother's room, a smaller angled shape for his and his brother's space, and a medium-sized shape to represent his sister's room. It seemed like a tight configuration. To demonstrate where his mother slept, he penciled in an area with a rectangular shape, which he called a couch, and smaller square shape that he denoted as a television.

He pointed out all these details in the picture to me and said, "This is the big room. My mother sleeps here on the couch."

When I asked him how often he stays at his grandmother's place, he put his finger on the picture and said, "We don't stay here a lot."

On a third piece of paper, he quickly executed a rectangular box shape. He drew three other boxes next to this shape. He said, "This is Jimmy's trailer. These are the four-wheelers." He showed me by putting his finger on the smaller box drawings.

I placed his drawings in front of him and smiled at the quality of his work. I understood from his visual depictions the impact divorce had on him. He slept in three different places. He was most comfortable at his father's. His grandmother's place was crowded. Jimmy's trailer seemed to be all about the four-wheelers.

I asked, "Do you know the visit schedule you have with your mother and father?"

He said, "I go to Mom's for some days, then I go to Dad's, but it always changes." He couldn't clearly articulate the three-day/four-day plan.

I noticed the time and let him know I was going to bring his mother in from the waiting area. He continued to be engaged in his drawings.

As his mother came into my office to be part of the intervention, he pointed to his Pokémon picture to show her, but his exuberance was immediately quelled, as his mother had her own agenda. She strode in, jaw tense, and before she even seated herself she asked, "Did you tell him about your father? Did you tell him your father doesn't spend time with you?"

He didn't respond but, instead, meekly looked up at his drawing on the bulletin board. She sat down on the couch. She followed his eyes to the drawing, relaxed a bit, and said, "You seem to always like to draw."

"I love Pokémon! That's the games I play." He pointed to his picture on the bulletin board and said, "See my drawing? It's a Pokémon. I colored it in."

She paid more attention to his production as he described the character with an abundance of detail. As he spoke, his mother's brown eyes widened in admiration. "Now I see why he plays those games for hours," she said.

I asked him if I could show his mother his other pictures. He nodded his head to show agreement. I wanted to see if his mother noticed anything about how he drew the places where he slept. She didn't seem to see anything particular in his visual interpretations. While Dominic drew and listened, I talked to her about the difficulties children of divorce have adjusting to different households and rules. I expressed to his mother that he displayed some confusion about the visitation schedule. "He couldn't explain the three-day/four-day plan to me," I said.

"I don't get how he has trouble with the schedule. I always tell him when it's time to go to his father's," she said. "His father probably doesn't do this."

Perhaps his strong visual comprehension could help him understand the visitation schedule. I explained to her that he needed more of an overview of the week. I suggested that she might want to set up a monthly calendar to help him visually identify which household he was scheduled to be at. I showed them a sample blank month from my appointment book. We talked about getting blank forms at the store.

He liked the concept. "I can draw on it. I can make Mom and Dad pictures."

His mother seemed to like the idea as well. She appeared slightly surprised, as I think she expected to talk more about the problems she suspected he had at his father's household. She believed his father didn't spend time with him. I didn't see this as a major concern. Divorced parents often compete over who provides the best home. I explained to her that my role would not be to talk about the other household with the parent who is not part of that household. However, if shared parenting rules needed to be established for the benefit of the child, such as consistent bedtimes, homework, or worries the child had, I would do that with both parents separately.

We concluded our time. Nicole had scheduled an appointment with Ruth for Mariah in a couple of weeks. I planned on contacting Gary to set up a first session for Bradley.

* * *

Bradley's rather bulky figure was easily identified as I approached him in the waiting area. As he glanced at his father, an imposing figure as well, he said, "So this is the doctor Dominic told me about." His father nodded his head. I brought Bradley into my office.

Bradley strategically sat in the middle of my couch so he was able to scan my entire office area. After a sigh of relief, he focused on the pictures displayed on the bulletin board. Pointing, he asked, "Is that Dominic's drawing?"

I smiled, as I watched the intensity of his interest without acknowledging any private details. I realized he must have talked with his brother about his time with me.

He responded with, "He told me to look for it. I can tell it's his. I know his drawings." He appeared to be reassured knowing that his brother had been in the office before him. He relaxed as he began to talk about himself. "I don't like Pokémon. That's Dominic's thing. I would rather ride four-wheelers."

I asked him, "How are you dealing with the different places you live in?" This spurred him to launch into recanting the past weekend he spent at Jimmy's trailer.

"I was riding the four-wheeler. We made a course in the woods. We built some awesome jumps," he stated. He clarified that he rode the four-wheelers with James and Evan—Jimmy's kids—and mostly stayed outside with them. I was curious if he knew what his brother and sister did while at the trailer. Bradley appeared excited telling me about riding motorized vehicles, and I wondered if he would have the same level of interest talking about his siblings.

About his brother, he said, "He doesn't like to ride, and he stays inside and plays his games. And Mariah—" He sat back on his seat and thought. "She's probably on her phone. She's always texting her friends."

I attempted to explore more about his interest in and knowledge of motorized vehicles. He spent some time going into detail about different types of four-wheelers. He then went back to reflecting on the past weekend. He described how he was able to repair one of the vehicles.

"Evan's four-wheeler wouldn't start," he stated. "I said maybe it was the spark plug. Of course, James said I didn't know what I was talking about. He thinks I'm stupid and never believes me. So I cleaned off the rusted plug, and it started. James told me it was luck."

After he contemplated for a short period, he shared, "I wish I had a four-wheeler at Dad's."

I told him this was something we could talk to his father about, as I saw it was getting near time for his father to be part of the session. I thought this would allow for a discussion around his interest and what his father would think about such a large purchase. He agreed to his father coming in. I said we could talk about four-wheelers and the divorce. I reminded him he was here because of his parents' divorce.

Gary positioned himself next to his son on the couch. Father and son sitting together visually established their physical resemblance to each other, as they were both hefty, imposing figures with large hands, dark eyes and hair, and quiet composure. I started by encouraging Bradley to talk about his interest in motorized vehicles with his father.

He talked about riding a four-wheeler and building a track in the woods at the trailer. His father listened to his adventures. Bradley looked at me and then looked at his father and asked him, "Can you get me a four-wheeler?" Then he repeated the question to his father, this time without making eye contact with him: "Can you get me a four-wheeler?"

Gary, in an almost emotionless manner, replied, "We talked about this already. As I recall, I told you we can't afford one now."

His son said, "I have one at Jimmy's."

"Is it yours?" his father asked him.

"No!" Bradley admitted. "It's James's old one."

Gary turned toward his son and for both our benefits asked, "Do you remember when we talked about how you could earn one?"

Looking downcast, Bradley replied, "Yeah, yeah, by doing chores and other jobs, I could earn money."

His father filled in the rest with, "After you've saved money, in maybe a year or so, I'd help you buy a four-wheeler."

To reinforce his father's parenting value, I said, "It's important to teach children about money and help them learn how to earn expensive items." Gary complained, "Jimmy and Nicole allow the kids to do what they want at their place. They have no rules."

I said, "I am more interested in how you parent. You and Nicole have different ways of parenting. If Bradley decides to become a parent, he can learn from both ways and choose which is best for him."

"I like rules," Gary said. "Children need to earn things. I worked all my life for what I have. As you probably already know, Jimmy got the trailer from his parents, and he doesn't work."

His son watched in adoration as his father spoke, and he smiled in acceptance. He did make one comment, which was, "Yeah, Mom does whatever Jimmy wants."

I understood that Gary worked hard and expected the same from his children. I did see a need for him to be more specific about how Bradley could earn a four-wheeler. I tried to engage them in discussing the plan more.

Bradley suggested setting up a hidden cashbox in his room. He could hide his earnings in the box. Gary agreed with the idea. He would develop chores for his son so he could earn money. As I listened, he and his son negotiated that when he turned twelve, the purchase of a motorized vehicle would be appropriate. The two of them reached a deal that the vehicle would be paid for by a combination of his savings and his birthday money. We concluded our session.

* * *

Over time I continued to meet with Dominic and Bradley. Nicole and Gary would bring them in separately. I made an effort to share parenting concerns between them. I would inform them about what I was going to tell the other parent. I began to establish communication between Nicole and Gary about the children through me.

I wanted to confer with Ruth to see how her work was going with Mariah. While Ruth and I were sitting at our common space in the practice offices having lunch, we took the time to review the case. We had been working with the children for almost six months.

Ruth told me, "Mariah has made significant progress in her individual treatment over the past several months. She has shown an improvement in her self-confidence and feels empowered. She requested a session next week with her mother. She wants to express her concerns about the divorce to her. She is prepared to tell her mother she doesn't like being at the trailer. She's bored. She wants to see her friends."

The following week, Ruth and I met again at our lunch spot to go over her session with Mariah and Nicole. We reheated bowls of leftover chicken soup that we'd brought from home and then sat at the table. Ruth poured herself a glass of water and recounted the session.

"Mariah told her mother she hates being at the trailer," Ruth said. "She said that's why she stays in her room texting her friends. She confronted her mother about her always being in the bedroom with Jimmy. She complained that they never spent any quality time together. She didn't understand why she just couldn't stay at her grandmother's."

Ruth told me that Nicole listened intently as Mariah complained about the limited time they spent together. She acknowledged her daughter's concerns about being isolated at the trailer but said she had been unaware of Mariah's concerns.

"Mariah also told her that James, Jimmy's oldest, was a brat and bossy and was especially mean to Dominic," Ruth said. "He doesn't let Dominic touch any of his stuff or ride the four-wheelers."

Could we help the parents begin to understand their children's needs? Could we help the parents communicate about their children's worries and develop common parenting strategies? Could we help the parents realize that being in separate households causes unique problems for children?

Ruth rinsed her bowl in the sink and thought more about what Mariah had said. Then she went on. Ruth believed she observed a parental shift in Nicole. "She appeared absolutely devastated by what Mariah told her. She said she wanted to think more about Mariah feeling lonely at the trailer. She apologized to Mariah for not spending time with her. Nicole complained that her own mother was never there for her when she was a teenager. She wanted to be there for Mariah."

* * *

In time I asked Gary if he could bring Kate in, since she was involved with the children and might have some important input. She came with Gary for one of my sessions with Dominic. Kate was a petite woman with a pleasant smile. Dominic confidently smiled at both of them when he came with me for another playtime. As he walked with me, he glanced backed at them to indicate that he felt safe. I could tell Kate appeared quite bewildered, as this was her first time in the office setting. She was unaware of the expectations.

However, Gary assured her by saying, "Dominic goes in first and then we go in after."

Dominic came into my office with a drawing agenda. He wanted to outline his new favorite Pokémon, called a Mega Mewtwo X. He stood near his usual drawing spot. "He looks like this!" He crouched with his hands bent like claws by his chest and said, "It is a rare legendary creature. It stands upright on two legs and looks like a cat."

He sat down at the drawing table and grabbed some sheets of paper and the container of colored pencils. He started sketching out his character. As he busily worked on his depiction, he seemed content. I thought this might be a good time to talk about some concerns. I asked him if the calendar helped him understand the visitation plan.

He said, "It does help." He hesitated and continued, "I leave it with Mom."

I asked, "Do you have one at your dad's?"

He said, "I don't have one there." As he looked up from his drawing, he said, "My friend, Garrett—he plays Pokémon. He wanted to play with me. He says he never knows which house I'm at." He sketched out his creature's long, catlike tail.

Dominic managed to complete most of his drawing as we continued. I realized that the split households added to his difficulty with getting together with his friends. He still had confusion around which home he would be at over the weekend. At his age, he couldn't coordinate a social engagement without the help of a parent. When it was time for his father and Kate to come in, I suggested that we could talk to them about social playdates.

Dominic wanted to be the one to bring them into my office. When he returned with Gary and Kate, he pointed to his drawings on the board. "See? Those are my pictures!" His father quizzically inspected the pictures and asked, "What are they, some kind of weird-looking animals?"

Kate said to Gary she had knowledge of Pokémon characters from her current experience as a para educator in a second-grade classroom. Dominic repositioned himself at the drawing table as Gary and Kate placed themselves on the couch. Gary, still focused on the pictures, slowly seemed to absorb his son's enthusiasm for the unusual characters.

I addressed Dominic's confusion around the visitation schedule. As I smiled at him, I informed his father and Kate that he was missing out on playing with his friend Garrett. I explained to them that he was unable to tell his friends when he is at which household. He doesn't remember the visit plan. I talked about his strong visual memory. I described to them the visually oriented calendar that he'd been using at his grandmother's home.

His father complained, "I never heard about the calendar." Gary and Kate agreed that the calendar sounded like a good plan.

Kate chimed in, "I can help him with his friend Garrett." She glanced empathetically at Dominic and said, "I think I know who your friend's mother is." She asked him, "When I picked you up at school the other day, was that Garrett with you?"

He responded with a loud, "Yeah!"

She continued, "Well, remember when Garrett got into the car, and his mother waved at me?" Kate said she'd known Garrett's mother for many years. She said, "The next time I see her, I'll talk to her about you and Garrett getting together."

Dominic looked pleased as he took the time from his drawing to look at her.

I reviewed the calendar concept again with Gary and Kate. I shared, "That's why it's so important that you and Nicole communicate. The calendar would be a helpful tool for Dominic to understand when he is with each parent so he can tell his friends." I went over and asked him if he wanted me to hang up his drawing. He did. I said, "Maybe the next time I see you, you will have had a playdate with Garrett."

Kate added, "I can assure you, he will have one."

The session ended.

* * *

At a later time, Nicole had heard Kate came into a session and asked Ruth if Jimmy could come to the next session with her. Nicole wanted to review Mariah's comments about the trailer and Nicole not spending time with her. Ruth and I talked about this and decided to run the meeting together as co-therapists. We wanted to present a unified approach and show them the importance of talking about the children's concerns about splitting their time between the two households.

I was the one who approached them in the waiting area. Ruth had settled herself in my office. I noticed Nicole and Jimmy sat close to each other on separate chairs. I introduced myself. Jimmy glared at me as I invited them into my office. I wondered if he was angry or anxious. Did he really want to come, or did he come because Nicole wanted him there?

I attempted to reduce the tension by pointing to Dominic's pictures, which were still displayed along with the many other children's drawings on the bulletin board. Nicole showed some comfort, as she was more familiar with the setting. She commented positively. She noted the quality of her son's drawing and placed herself on the couch.

Jimmy was slightly taller than her and had followed her into the office. He sat next to her. Immediately he began to shift his position by sitting up stiff and straight. This physically accentuated his presence in the room. His face began to turn redder as he leered at Nicole and Ruth. He couldn't remain subdued anymore. I thought he really didn't want to come.

He stated, "So, what goes on in here?" He stared at Ruth and said, "We never had problems until you got involved." Nicole slithered slightly lower than him in her seat as he continued to protest.

He said, "Mariah is refusing to come to the trailer. She said you said it was okay."

Ruth encouraged Nicole to reflect on the session she had with her and her daughter. She asked, "Nicole, do you remember what we talked about with Mariah?"

Nicole remained focused on Ruth as she said, "Mariah made the decision on her own not to come over to the trailer. She said she was bored and wanted to see her friends. She felt stuck at the trailer. She said I never spent any time with her."

Jimmy turned his head toward Nicole and shot her a glance. I realized he was anxious about being a parent and didn't understand what was best to do. After gathering some sense of composure, he fumed, "Let Mariah do what she wants, I don't care. She never talks to us anyway. She hides in the back room talking to her friends on her cell phone." Loosening up and sliding down in his seat, he added, "If the kids don't care about the trailer and riding the four-wheelers, they don't have to come. My boys come every other weekend. It gets to be a lot of kids at times. It's only a small three-bedroom trailer."

Ruth had strategically made Mariah's point. Jimmy couldn't blame her. After that, he appeared not to be as angry. I understood from him that having all the children at the small trailer was difficult. I asked, "How do the two of you handle the children at the trailer?"

Jimmy described a belief in being more hands-off: "I don't mind if the boys spend the day riding the four-wheelers in the woods. They don't bother us. They get their own food if they need some." Nicole listened and didn't disagree.

Ruth delved more into their noninvasive approach to parenting from concerns we gathered from the children. She asked if they had any concerns about Dominic's and Mariah's eating alone in their rooms. It was not easy for Jimmy to talk about the children. He seemed to become irritated when we tried to discuss family issues. He didn't seem to want to comment about how to parent Nicole's children.

Nicole stated, "We don't have set mealtimes. The kids are old enough to get food for themselves. Sometimes we eat together when we cook out in the summer."

To this exchange, Jimmy seemed to become anxious again and stood up. He said, "It's time to go." He looked at Nicole. "She's a good mother; she knows what's best for the children."

He was right that the time was almost up. I told them that their input was helpful for the children's treatment. "Having all the children at the trailer sounds like a lot," I said. I suggested maybe Nicole and Gary could have another look at the visitation plan. Nicole said that the session was helpful.

Jimmy politely agreed. He said, "I said what I needed to say. The kids can come over whenever they want. It's up to Nicole. Whatever she wants."

I opened the door as I reminded Nicole that we would contact her to set up the next appointment.

Ruth and I spent some time processing the family issues in my office after they left. We talked about the backstory to Jimmy and Nicole's relationship. Ruth remembered what Nicole had said when Mariah complained that she didn't like Jimmy. "Nicole said Jimmy had been emotionally damaged by his parents' death in a car accident when he was in his early twenties. He inherited the land and trailer after their death. Jimmy told her he never wanted to be part of a family again."

We accepted that Jimmy had no interest in being a parental figure and wouldn't want to be part of developing a postdivorce family plan for Nicole and Gary's family. However, he seemed to respect Nicole's decision. The children were expressing their needs more, and the parents were listening.

Ruth said, "Mariah's honesty with her mother helped. She told her mother she had a boyfriend. She saw him when she stayed at her grandmother's. Her mother was upset about the lack of supervision. Nicole encouraged her to use birth control. She told her she didn't want her to become a pregnant teen like she had been. Nicole restated that she wanted to be there for her unlike her own mother had been for her. Mariah was appreciative of her mother's concerns."

* * *

A month or so later, Gary requested a parent session for him and Kate. He said on the phone he was confused about some recent developments. I scheduled an appointment so we could talk in more depth about what had occurred. I would meet with them alone and inform Ruth about their concerns.

They were used to office procedures and were on time. They sat comfortably next to each other on the couch in my office.

Gary opened the session with, "Nicole stopped me at the school pickup and said she was worried about Mariah."

I noticed that he seemed puzzled. I wondered if this was because he wasn't used to Nicole talking to him about any of the children. Kate appeared surprised as well. "That's unusual," I said. "What was her concern?"

"She said Mariah was staying at her grandmother's. She was apparently having her friends and boyfriend there. She was refusing to go to the trailer. Nicole was concerned about the lack of supervision at her mother's."

I observed his astonished look. Gary and Nicole had never shared concerns about their children like this before.

He looked at Kate and turned toward me and said, "I honestly didn't know how to respond. I told her I was going to make an appointment with you. I told her I would get back to her."

"Do you agree with her concerns?" I asked. I began to think this may be an opening to encourage more open communication between them about their children.

He said, "I am concerned because Nicole's mother is very ill. She has difficulty hearing. She stays in her bedroom watching television. The kids tell me the TV is loud. I don't think she can provide adequate supervision for a teenager. She has many medical issues and requires her own supervision."

Kate suggested, "Maybe Mariah could stay at our house. We could provide better supervision. I'm home every day after school. On weekends we're always around. Since we're in town, she can visit her friends. We can set up a curfew and rules."

"Sounds like some good ideas," I said. I asked Gary about the visitation agreement. Could he and Nicole make changes, if necessary?

He said, "We have joint decision-making and custody. We can make changes to the visitation schedule if we agreed."

I proposed that maybe he and Nicole could come up with a plan to address Mariah's need for adequate supervision. We had met with everyone in the family many times, but not with Nicole and Gary together. I asked if he would be willing to be in a session with Nicole, Ruth, and me. He said after his last interaction with Nicole, he might be prepared for such a joint session. I said I would let Ruth know what we discussed and contact Nicole. We ended the session.

* * *

I had a pleasant phone conversation with Nicole. "I would be willing to set up a better visit plan," she said. Later in the call, she added, "The lawyers mostly set up the agreement. I had become so tired of court. I just wanted it to end. I'm sick of still having to make payments to my lawyer." She gave me some potential times for a parent session.

We arrived at a common appointment time for the parents. Ruth and I had devised a strategy where we would each meet with one of the parents alone first. After that, the four of us would meet together. I decided to meet with Nicole, and Ruth would engage Gary.

We had a purpose for meeting alone with each parent. We wanted to help them sort out some possible visitation arrangements. This would avoid potential conflicts when we would meet together. Our goal would be to maintain their focus on the children's best interests and their needs. We hoped that, by helping each of them think through the concerns first, we could better work with them in learning to communicate with each other.

Ruth started off the combined intervention by saying, "The visitation plan doesn't currently address the interests of the children." She encouraged Nicole to explain what she thought would work best.

Nicole said, "I think it would be better if the children came over every other weekend when Jimmy's boys weren't there. This would make the trailer less crowded. Jimmy would like this. And I would have more time with them. I would like Mariah to stay at least one night at the trailer. She could spend the other night at his place." She looked over at Gary and briefly made eye contact. She continued, "The next day, I would like to have some alone time with her."

Gary responded positively and said, "I'm okay with some of the changes you're talking about. I think I need to talk with Kate."

Ruth suggested, "Why don't you each present what arrangements you think would work best for the children? We can then sort through them. Do you want to continue?" she asked Nicole.

Nicole continued, "I'd like to have one or two overnights during the school week at my mother's home. I want to be able to see my children when I'm not at the trailer. This three-day/four-day schedule doesn't work."

Gary agreed: "I don't like it either. It doesn't work for me or the kids."

I asked if they had thought about school vacations. I had already brought up the idea of splitting the vacation time when I met with Nicole.

The parents cordially consented to splitting the vacations. By this time they were making eye contact with each other and having a productive conversation. They managed to develop a plan about vacations. The concept they discussed was that whoever had the children for the weekend before vacation would just have the children remain in that household until mid-week.

Ruth asked Nicole, "Do you realize that Dominic said he has no interest in riding the four-wheelers at the trailer? He said he wanted to have more playtime with friends."

"I'm starting to get that our children have their own needs," Nicole said. She looked at Gary and gave him a small smile. "I want to figure out how we can change some of the schedule for them. I am worried about my mother. She seems to require more care. She can't watch the children and supervise them."

Gary said, "We can help as much as possible. I don't think your mother should be left alone with the children."

I was impressed that both parents could address the concerns about the visitation agreement and endorse several mutual changes. They still had distrust of each other. But they were learning to establish a productive dialogue and a positive manner of communication around the best interests of the children. Our therapeutic work was to keep the focus on the children. The children wanted to please each parent. Therefore Gary and Nicole tended to hear different concerns. We encouraged them to be mindful of what would benefit the children.

After several sessions and consultations with their significant others, Gary and Nicole produced a new visitation arrangement. We had a final meeting to review the document. In general, the agreement allowed more flexibility. The children didn't go to the trailer when Jimmy's children were there. A summer barbecue at Jimmy's could be arranged in advance. Dominic was able to have friends over. Mariah stayed at her father's but had time alone with her mother. Both parents agreed to communicate more directly about the children. They would keep each other informed about school and medical appointments. The plan was completed, and copies were submitted to their attorneys.

Nicole and Gary left our office with a deeper understanding of how divorce breaks up a family into two factions and separates the family into households. Their marital conflicts had affected their ability to communicate and talk about the individual needs of their children. Over time, as split parents, they began to realize that decisions around visitation had to take account of their children's needs. In order to establish postdivorce communication, they had to work on not letting their personal issues get in the way of what was in the best interests of their children.

CHALLENGES AND REFLECTIONS

The challenge of this divorce case was to keep the focus on the children. Dominic's drawings helped me understand the differences in the households he lived in. I was able to see his family through his keen visual perspective. This was different from what Nicole originally presented. Gary attempted to be a caring parent and listened to the children.

As co-therapists, Ruth and I included Gary and Nicole in their children's treatment. The children expressed their concerns in therapy. Dominic shared his interest in visual activities. He missed having playdates with his friends. This was complicated by him living in two different places. Bradley liked riding the motorized vehicles at Jimmy's trailer. This caused conflicts when Jimmy's children would visit. Mariah had teenage plans. She didn't like being at either of her parents' homes. She wanted time with her friends. In parenting sessions, Ruth and I helped Nicole and Gary understand their children's concerns and worries.

Ruth had a challenging session with Mariah and Nicole. Mariah had the courage to tell her mother about her feelings. She didn't like living in two different homes. This was a turning point in our treatment. It helped Nicole understand the problem of divorce. She became aware that the lack of any positive interactions between her and Gary caused problems.

This knowledge spurred Nicole and Gary to work together as parents. As co-therapists, Ruth and I helped them change their visitation arrangements. We helped them revise their parenting strategies. They communicated with each other about the needs of their children. They put aside their anger to support their children.

Chapter 7

Arty's Secret Winner

PRESENTING PROBLEMS

Arty, a twelve-year-old boy, was a product of a dysfunctional family. Sherry, his mother, had severe psychiatric and emotional problems. Art, his father, was an alcoholic. Misty, a close family friend, brought Arty in for therapy. She presented his history. She understood his sadness. Misty wanted him to get help.

Sherry and Arty lived in Misty's home. She provided a stable household for them. Arty was resistant to treatment. He felt like he didn't have any parents. He felt uncared for. He talked about feeling lonely. He mistrusted adults. Arty struggled with these issues throughout his treatment. In adolescence, he was placed in a residential facility. His behavior had become risky and dangerous. Misty remained loyal and committed to him. He realized how much she cared for him. Misty became his secret winner.

TREATMENT STORY

"Hello, my name is Misty, and I'm calling about a twelve-year-old boy who needs counseling."

This message on my answering machine suggested that Misty might not be asking about her own child, so when I returned Misty's call, I asked if she was the parent or guardian of the boy she called about. When she confessed that she was not, I explained that in order for me to treat a child I had to have consent from a legal guardian or parent.

Misty explained the situation. She said Arty and his mother, Sherry, lived with her in her apartment. Sherry was recently discharged from a psychiatric hospital. One of the recommendations was for her to have her son, Arty, go to counseling.

I asked if I could hear from Sherry, and Misty handed over the phone. Sherry got on and said, simply, "Arty needs counseling. I can't drive. Misty has to take him." She offered no further explanation. Before I could follow up, she had already given the phone back to Misty. I figured that would have to do and coordinated a time to meet with Misty and Sherry for an initial intake to authorize treatment. After gathering family information at this session, I would set up a meeting with Arty.

* * *

On the day of the appointment, I was surprised to find not two but three women seated in the waiting room. A young, energetic woman jumped up and, clasping my hand, introduced herself as Libby, Sherry's counselor. She said she was here to assist the boy's mother with the paperwork.

Next to Libby was a slightly obese woman with gray-streaked hair. She remained slumped in her chair and stared blankly at the counselor. I surmised this was Sherry, as she had the lack of connection that can be associated with severe emotional illness. I believed because of her puffy-faced appearance that she might be on a high dose of psychiatric medication. I thought this was probably the case as she was recently discharged from the hospital.

The third woman intently watched the interactions while leaning forward in her seat on a walking stick. She was slightly heavy, with short, evenly cut hair; she sported a distinguished, tan-colored dress. She smiled politely at me and introduced herself as Misty. I handed the clipboard with its packet of forms to the boy's mother, who in turn slid it over to the counselor. I went back to my office to give them time to complete the paperwork.

When I came back to the waiting room, Libby stood up and handed me the completed packet. I asked Sherry if she was comfortable with the others accompanying her into the session. She signaled her consent by slowly nodding.

Once in my office, the three of them placed themselves on my long couch with the boy's mother sitting in the middle. Looking at the three of them, I said I needed to learn more about Arty's problems. Why did he require counseling? Why was this part of the discharge suggestion for Sherry? I also wanted to establish that the purpose of our meeting was Arty's treatment.

Sherry responded with a series of distressed statements: "He doesn't care. He does what he wants. Nobody can stop him. He hides in his room. He's mean, like his dad." With a sigh of exasperation and some tears, she concluded, "I just don't get it." Libby gave her a supportive look while Misty held her hand to comfort her.

I thanked her for sharing her concerns and asked for more information about Arty's family situation.

Misty said, "I'm like his step-grandparent." Eyeing Sherry, she continued, "Arty and his mother share my three-bedroom apartment. I work as a book-keeper for a local physician. I'm Sherry's payee for her disability checks. This income helps pay the rent for her and Arty."

Libby edged herself into the conversation. "She has these benefits because of her severe depression," she said. "She gets no help from his father, Art."

I didn't want to exclude Libby's opinions, but I needed to hear more about Arty's family concerns. I asked if Misty could explain how she had become involved with the family.

Misty said, "Sherry and my daughter, Lacey, were best friends in high school. When Lacey died from an overdose, Sherry and I helped each other through the grief. Lacey was our only child. Walt, my husband, never got over it, and he died several years later. Sherry and I became very close. Then she got involved with Art. He was a top-notch mechanic and fixed cars in his yard. He helped repair my car many times. But then he became involved with Candy, his current girlfriend. She turned him into a drunk."

I thought Misty might have the clearest grasp of Arty's early years. She was not pleased by the boy's father's choices, and it was clear she didn't approve of Candy. But I needed to determine the effect of both the father's drinking and the mother's illness on the boy. "How did they end up living with you?" I asked.

Misty continued, "I told her she couldn't trust Art. She ended up getting pregnant by him. She finally left him after Arty was born. I don't think she ever got over him. I took them in, and then we moved to a larger place." Misty turned her head toward Sherry and asked, "Are you okay with what I said?" Sherry said she was.

"Can anyone shed some light on the boy's relationship with Art?" I asked. I looked at Sherry. I didn't expect an answer from her, as she appeared dis-engaged and nonresponsive, but I wanted to try to keep her attention. When Sherry didn't answer, I looked toward Misty and asked, "What about Arty and Art's relationship?"

"I can tell you I never liked him after he became involved with Candy," Misty responded. "He became real nasty the more he drank. Threatening his customers, saying horrible things to people. I heard people started calling him 'Darth' behind his back—you know, like Darth Vader. I thought it was about right. I stopped bringing my car to him. The more he drank, the nastier he became, and the more people called him Darth." Misty turned to Sherry. "Isn't that right, Sherry?" Sherry looked at her as if in agreement.

"Does the boy see his father much?" I asked.

Misty said, "He visits his dad as little as possible. He has no respect for him. That man only lives for his drinking. Darth couldn't care less for his son, and I'm afraid Arty knows it. He told me his dad is mean." As she turned toward Sherry with a sad look in her eyes, she added, "Art left this woman and her baby at birth."

Sherry, who had nearly fallen asleep, perked up a little at these statements.

I wanted to gather more about Arty's early development. Each of his parents had significant problems. I now realized why treatment was recommended for the boy. I assumed that Misty was going to be the most accurate reporter to discuss his upbringing. His mother seemed to have tuned out, and at times, I noticed her head bobbed with her eyes closed.

"Arty had problems from the beginning," Misty said. "His mother was hospitalized when he was around six months old."

The counselor interrupted her. "You know that was the first of many other psychiatric hospitalizations," Libby asserted as she looked at me. "I reviewed the report. The evaluation concluded Sherry was at serious risk of harming herself; she was severely depressed, she refused to eat, and she wouldn't leave her bedroom. She required immediate hospitalization."

Sherry opened her eyes and seemed saddened. I asked her how she was doing. She made eye contact with me and said, "Good." To refocus the intake on Arty, I encouraged Misty to present more of the history.

Misty started where she left off. "I had to call the Rescue Squad. She had been in bed for several days, and the smell was awful. She wouldn't move or respond to me. She was brought to the hospital for a psychiatric evaluation. I took care of the baby while all this was going on."

"How were Arty's early school years?" I asked, still trying to refocus on Arty.

Misty looked at Sherry and said, "I helped her register Arty for preschool. Since I had the car, I arranged my schedule so I could take him to school and pick him up. I would also take time to talk to his teachers."

"What did his teachers say about his behavior?" I began to realize the significant place Misty had in Arty's development. She had assumed the role of his primary caretaker.

Misty said, "I recall his first- and second-grade teachers saying he was a good learner. They said he had an endearing quality. But he had some days where he wouldn't listen, or he'd sometimes antagonize his peers. Other times he would completely shut down."

"Do you have any idea why the boy would isolate himself, be aggressive, or shut down?" Since Arty was now twelve, I was curious if over the years Misty had noticed a pattern to his behavior. Did he act unpredictably, or were there external circumstances for his actions? If Misty could explain this, I would have some beginning therapeutic goals for Arty.

She said, "I eventually figured it out. Arty's acting out happened after he had a visit with his father. It was always at the beginning of the week on a weekend after he saw Darth."

I believed Misty might be right on. It made sense that he'd be impacted by his father's actions. I was interested if she could describe what his interactions with his father were like. "Did Arty ever tell you about what went on at his father's household?" I asked.

"He told me a little. He told me Art would call him stupid and make fun of him and his mother. He told me Darth said Sherry was mental and crazy." Misty glanced at Sherry, but she didn't appear to be listening. "He said Art said he should live with him. Darth told him his mother and I were both nuts."

"What happened at home when he returned from his father's?" I believed if Arty was affected by his father's actions that she would notice this after he returned.

"He would hide in his room. I would come in to see how he was doing, and he'd be crying and upset. I think he was in third grade when he told me the truth about how bad the visits were. I couldn't take seeing the child so sad and hurt. I decided something had to be done."

"Were you able to do anything about the visitation?" I asked. Misty was not the custodial parent, and Sherry had significant problems. It would have been quite an undertaking for her to take the case to family court.

Misty explained, "I persuaded Sherry to go to court with me. I helped her change the agreement. Art never contested. He didn't even show up. He ended up with no rights."

Libby added, "I am working with Misty to help her obtain legal guardianship."

I thanked Libby for her support. I smiled at Sherry and said to Misty that the information she provided was helpful for my understanding of the family issues. Obviously, I had concerns about the destructive nature of the boy's relationship with his father. I believed Arty might not have inherited his mother's condition, since he apparently had some awareness of his behavior and didn't become sad and depressed. Misty confirmed this—he did have an awareness of his actions. I was worried about the effect of his father's rejecting criticisms. I scheduled an appointment for Arty with Misty. She agreed to bring Sherry and Arty.

* * *

Misty arrived promptly with Arty and Sherry for this next session. I had a feeling she would be responsible and reliable. Arty was looking at a children's magazine when I entered the waiting room. He was a slightly obese boy with sad green eyes. He had on a nice pair of Carhartt slacks and shirt. Sherry was slumped in the same chair she had sat in before. Misty introduced the boy to me and encouraged him to go with me into my office. "He has a lot more toys and games in his office," she said. Listening to her reassurance, the child followed me without resistance.

Noticing the playthings in my office, he appeared interested. I asked, "Would you like to play a game?"

He said, "I play checkers with my dad." I pulled the checkers game off the shelf and placed the board on the play table to set up the game. Grabbing the black pieces, he stated, "I can beat anyone."

When arranging the black checkers pieces, he placed them on the white squares. I gently let him know that this wasn't how we usually play. "When we play, we usually place the checkers on the black squares."

"Forget it!" he said. "You don't know what you're talking about." Pushing the game away, he added, "I don't want to play."

I put the game away. I decided to try another game in order to ease his agitation. I pulled out the Uno cards. I began shuffling the deck numerous times in a rhythmical manner. He watched closely, somewhat mesmerized. I asked if he played. He said he did, and I asked him how many cards I should deal out. I wanted to see if I could involve him in the game. I wanted him to make a decision.

"Six," he said.

I dealt out six cards each. We established the rules of play. We agreed to play three games. The winner would be defined as the first to win two games. We played "Rock, Paper, Scissors" to determine who would go first. I was hoping he would win. Happily, he did.

He committed himself to the match. He seemed calmer and more accepting.

Before Arty made his first move, he carefully looked through the cards in his hand. He placed two cards down cunningly to the side. I asked, "What are those cards for?"

He glanced at my eyes for the first time and responded, "They are my secret winners."

Interspersed during our card play, I was able to tease out some critical information. He informed me that the only reason he went to school was to see his friends. He complained that he didn't like to do homework.

Throughout the game, he would add more cards to his secret stash. Finally, I reminded him I only had a couple more cards left, and I was ready to win the game. It was his turn. Uncovering his coveted pile of cards, he proceeded to place one winning card after another until he won.

As I shuffled the cards for our next game, I asked him about visiting his father. "What do you do when you go over to your father's?"

"I like helping him fix cars," he said.

"Misty told me he has a drinking problem." I wanted to understand how he dealt with his father's alcoholism.

He seemed to feel he had some control over the relationship, as he insisted, "I leave when we're done working on the cars and he goes into the house. I don't like when him and Candy sit and drink. I say I have to go home."

I asked him about his mother, and he told me, "She's always in her room watching TV. She only comes out to smoke." His voice sounded sadder than before.

"What about Misty?" I asked.

"I call her Gammy," he said. He pointed to his new sneakers, pants, and shirt and said, "Gammy got me these." I asked him if he had ever been to a counselor before, and he shook his head. "Gammy always wants me to go."

I dealt out the Uno cards again. He used the same strategy of putting some cards in his secret stash. Eventually he used these winning cards to beat me for the second time and won the match. I asked, "Are you ready for your mother and Gammy to be part of the session?" I explained that I like to include parents and significant other adults.

He consented to this plan, but first he had a question. "How do you mix the cards?" he asked. I showed him how to halve the deck and place his thumbs on top of each half and let the cards go so he could shuffle them. He tried it and managed to do it. I said I was going out to the waiting room to get his mother and Misty. He said he wanted to stay in my office. "I want to practice shuffling the cards."

His mother came into the treatment room first and slowly maneuvered herself into the large chair. Misty, a rather large woman herself, hobbled in with the assistance of her walking stick. Surveying the space, she placed herself on the couch closer to where the boy was sitting. Once she settled in her seat, she commanded the conversation.

Peering directly at the boy she said, "I really want Arty to get some help. If he doesn't get help, I worry he's going to have big problems." He turned toward her, and she looked directly at him as she went on. "He's a good child. I care very much about him." Turning her gaze toward me, she said, "What I am going to say he already knows. There are times when he does what he wants. Times when he doesn't care. Times when he seems to have no morals. Times when he doesn't listen to his teachers. He has no goals. The worst is the times he only looks to do no good." Her tone was assertive but empathetic.

I noticed the boy intently listening. His mother seemed alert as well.

"This is what I worry about," Misty continued, picking up her walking stick to gesture with. She turned toward the boy and said, "The major problem he has is his father. That man is a piece of work. Arty should not visit him. He has let Candy take over his life."

"What exactly do you think is the problem with his father?" I asked. I hoped Misty could clearly describe her worries.

"Arty knows his dad hasn't been sober enough to get what a good son he has. When Arty sees him, he drinks. He becomes mean and says hurtful comments to him about his mother. I ask myself, how much can this boy take?"

"I leave when he starts getting drunk," Arty reminded her.

The boy and his mother had been keenly watching Misty's performance. Both seemed to be in awe as she held onto her walking stick while she talked. This dramatization accentuated her status in the family.

* * *

Over time, Misty followed through on bringing Arty and his mother to treatment. Arty continued to become more engaged in therapy. He enjoyed playing Uno. His secret winner strategy was usually successful. He had learned to shuffle the deck. He started to trust the relationship enough to share some of his concerns. He occasionally had visits with his father, and he continued to say that he always left when it got to be too much. He expressed fears related to his father's alcoholism. He hated his father's rejecting comments. And he worried about his mother's severe depressive illness. He didn't understand what was the matter with her.

Arty, in time, began to realize his mother was sad and depressed, and she needed medicine to help her. Sometimes she couldn't help being very unhappy for no reason. He continued to visit his father and enjoyed learning about repairing cars. He always made sure to leave before his father became too drunk.

* * *

After about a year of treatment, I came into the office one morning when Arty had a scheduled appointment. I checked the answering machine and saw that someone had left a message at 3 a.m. It was Misty. The message was unusually brief for her: "I can't get him to the appointment."

After several missed attempts, I finally was able to contact her late that afternoon. She told me that Sherry had swallowed her bottle of pills and was hospitalized. She apologized for not being able to make the appointment and said she would speak to me at a later time. She immediately ended the call.

About a week later, Misty requested an appointment. I left a message on her cell phone suggesting a scheduled time. I asked her to contact me if they were unable to attend.

I entered the waiting room at the planned time, expecting to accompany Arty into my office. Instead, Misty was seated there by herself. She looked at me sadly and said, "I'm sorry. I need to talk to you."

* * *

I escorted her into my office, and she eased herself on the couch with the help of her cane. "Sherry has been placed in the inpatient unit," she said. "She has been labeled as severely depressed. I was told she may be there for several weeks. She hasn't responded to the new medication."

I thought this must be upsetting for both her and the boy. So why hadn't Arty come? He was probably struggling with his mother's attempt to harm herself. He must need to process the situation. I asked her, "Where is Arty?"

"Well, I am going to tell you why Arty is not here. When his mother was at the unit, Arty decided to walk over to his father's. I expected him to be home for dinner when I returned from the hospital. It never happened. Instead, a police officer contacted me and said he was at the station. He told me Arty was in state's custody. So I went over there, and Arty was in tears. He said to me in the presence of an officer that his father was drunk. He said his father wouldn't stop making comments about his mother, calling her the crazy lady."

I realized the gravity of the situation: Arty's mother in hospital after attempting suicide, and Arty himself in custody at the police station. I was worried about Arty. I asked Misty to please continue her story.

"I think with his mother in the hospital, Arty reacted differently to his father's nasty comments about her. He apparently ran out of his father's apartment with his father's loaded gun. He proceeded to kill a neighbor's cat. He was shooting at birds when the police arrived."

So that was why the boy was placed in state's custody. He had engaged in violent juvenile activity with a weapon. This was an extreme level of dangerous behavior for Arty. It wasn't usual for him. He would probably be placed in a foster home until his risk level was assessed. "Have you been in contact with his state social worker?" I asked Misty.

Her cane began to shake in her hand. Misty, who rarely lost her composure, appeared devastated by the events. After a moment, she said, "The social worker has already contacted me. I'm the boy's legal guardian and have a joint custodial arrangement with his mother. She said Arty would eventually be back in my household."

"I'm sorry," I said. "It sounds like you have a lot to handle. Arty's actions were dangerous. You and I know he has a good heart. He must have been deeply hurt." I went on, "The legal process may take some time, but hopefully Arty will be placed in your home with conditions." I asked, "How can I help?"

She said, "Arty is going to be on probation. I want him to continue seeing you for counseling. I think he likes you. I don't believe he's a violent kid. He just needs help and someone he can talk to."

We set up a plan where she would keep me in the loop. I told her I was committed to seeing Arty for therapy. Arty would remain in foster care until the juvenile court hearings were completed and he was not a serious risk for committing other violent acts. I explained to her that the state had legal custody, and the court matters would take about six months. He would then be placed back in her home. I encouraged her to work with the state social worker.

* * *

Arty's treatment during those six months became sporadic due to the limitations of the foster care system he was in. Misty made every effort she could.

But Child Protective Services had trouble finding a placement for an almost fourteen-year-old boy who was deemed at risk to be violent. He was placed in several different foster homes and eventually ended up in a home about an hour away.

When he attended therapy, we played Uno and talked. He missed his family, especially his Gammy. He admitted he felt lonely, sad, and frustrated with not being home. His risk had been assessed. A recommendation was made for him to stay away from his father. He told me he felt consumed by his anger at his father. He felt bad about his aggression toward animals. We wrote a letter of apology together to the cat's owner. His words showed compassion. I believed he wasn't at risk of harming himself or others. He just wanted to be home. This became the goal of Child Protective Services.

Misty was extremely frustrated with the legal system. It took more than six months before Arty was reunified with his family. She believed that the placement was on hold due to Sherry's relapse and suicide attempts. The state's attorney had to review her psychiatric history. They questioned her competency to parent. Fortunately, Misty was established as the primary caregiver. Arty was placed at her home before the holidays of his freshman year of high school.

* * *

Arty attended a session during that Christmas vacation. Misty brought him. His mother didn't come. He was dressed in a new outfit and sneakers. When he came into my office, he had no interest in playing our usual card game. He wanted to talk. I asked, "How is your mother doing?"

He said, "She sits in her bedroom in her nightclothes. I don't think she even knew I was in another home. I tried to explain to her what happened to me. She didn't seem to understand."

Misty had already provided me with the recent court order. Arty was only supposed to visit his father if he was sober. I realized this was going to be difficult to monitor. I believed his father probably wouldn't be able to follow through on the order and not drink. I asked Arty what he thought of this plan.

He smirked and said, "Whatever that means. I don't want to see him anyway. Nobody can make me. I don't have to see him if I don't want to."

We talked about how happy he was to finally be home. Arty was unclear about his home placement and probation condition. I asked if we could bring Misty in as she might be better able to explain his legal circumstances. He agreed. I left the office to bring her in from the waiting room.

Leaning on her walking stick, she took her favorite spot on the couch next to the boy. Once she was positioned, I informed her that Arty didn't understand his current legal situation.

Knowledgeable as usual, Misty said, "Arty is in state's custody but placed at our household. He has to continue to follow his conditions. He has to attend school, pass his classes, continue in therapy, and not get in any more trouble. If he does that, custody will be returned to his mother and me after about three months." She wiggled her cane as she smiled at Arty.

I asked if Arty understood the rules. "If you do what you are supposed to the state will be out of your life."

He said, "I get it."

Misty added, "His mother was unable to come today. She's on a new medication. She has no ability to help me with Arty. It's all up to me." She turned toward Arty but continued talking to me. "I will be honest with you. He didn't want to come today. He told me he doesn't need it. His probation officer told him he had to come. You know Arty doesn't like to be told what to do."

Arty said nothing in response. Nevertheless, he committed to continue coming. He knew it was one of his required probation conditions.

* * *

Over the next several months, Arty reluctantly came to his sessions. Misty provided the ride. His mother occasionally attended. When she came, she offered minimal input. At one point, she began muttering to herself during a family session. Arty seemed to be accustomed to this type of behavior from his mother and acted as if he didn't notice.

In time, I began to see a darker side of Arty in treatment. His peer group and new girlfriend were into partying and drugs. He talked about dropping out of school. He struggled to follow his probation conditions.

Eventually Misty shared in a family session that they had had their final court hearing the previous week and Arty had been placed at her home. "He still has to continue with probation," she said. "He wants to drop out of school. He said he doesn't want to come to counseling anymore."

I asked Arty what he thought of Misty's comments. I mentioned that he couldn't legally drop out of school until he was sixteen. I also reminded him that counseling was a condition of his probation.

"Okay, I will stay in school," Arty said. "But I know older kids who have dropped out and are working. They have a car and money."

Misty said, "As long as you are living in my home, I want you to complete high school. You can drop out at sixteen, but you have to get a GED. I can accept you working, but you need to finish high school in some way. You told me you don't want to be like your father. Well, he never finished school and he doesn't have a real job."

Arty listened to Misty's demands. She accepted his concerns about school. I believed Arty was still tormented by his parents' inadequacies. He had intense anger toward his father. His mother's severe depression incapacitated her. She could barely function. His potential to abuse substances and act out his anger was still high. He had no goals and was involved with a risky peer group. I tried my best to reach him in therapy, but I had difficulty overcoming his resistance. I told him my worries. He said he only came because he had to come. However, once he was in my office he was able to open up.

* * *

Then, on the day of one of our sessions, Misty left a disturbing message: "Sherry is in the hospital. She overdosed and took all her medication again. I can't bring Arty today."

When we connected by phone after a couple of weeks, she was quite upset. She complained that Arty had refused to go to school. She told me, "I'm done. I can't do this anymore."

Arty had become even more defiant. He was not respecting Misty's authority. He wasn't following his legal conditions. I thought he may need to be placed in a more secure facility. I shared my concerns. Misty responded, "I haven't been able to reach him. I think he's doing drugs. His probation officer called me. He hasn't shown up for his mandatory meeting. She said she is going to violate him." She requested an appointment for her and Arty.

On the planned visit, Misty sat alone in the waiting area. When I asked her about Arty, she shook her head and said, "He won't be coming today." After hobbling her way with her walking stick through the office door, she found her comfort seat.

Misty appeared unusually frustrated. Her hand couldn't stop trembling while holding her cane. I hadn't seen this look from her. She was the source of strength in the family. This time her expression was of defeat and sadness. I could tell she was heartbroken. I needed to approach her sensitively. I asked her about the situation.

She said, "I can't handle the boy. He refuses to listen to me. I think he's on drugs. He steals money from me. He's not the same Arty I cared so much about. We can't talk anymore. Everything is a fight and argument."

I knew his blatant refusal to come to therapy today was a problem. He had become completely oppositional. He couldn't even talk to Misty.

Misty said, "He told me therapy never helped his mother. I tried to explain that his mother has severe depression. He said he didn't care. He wasn't going to counseling. He didn't need it. I can't tell him what to do, he told me." She managed to hold her cane still. "His mother attends a daily treatment program. At least they transport her. The rest of the time she stays in her bedroom. But Arty scares me. He makes threats about hurting his father. He doesn't see him. He has no relationship with his mother. He used to sit with her in her room. Now he's never around. He's always out, and I don't know where he is. He won't listen to me."

Arty did not respect her or any authority. I encouraged her to explain her concerns to his probation officer. I suggested that he may need a more intensive level of supervision. I told her I would contact his probation officer as well.

She said, "I was feeling all alone. Thanks for talking. I feel better. I just want Arty to get help. He must feel all alone, too." As she left my office, she said she would keep me updated.

* * *

A mandate from his probation officer ordered him to attend a final session. He had just turned sixteen. He was being placed in a residential facility. Misty brought him to our final meeting. It was not productive. He sat in the corner of the waiting room; his head was down with his hands covering his forehead. He came into my office without looking at me.

I attempted to engage him after he sat on the couch. "I'm sorry to hear about your placement. The Keene faculty you are going to can be helpful. You will get your high school diploma and job skills."

But he didn't want to hear what I had to say. He stood up and said, "This counseling is stupid! I'm done with it!" He abruptly left and slammed my office door.

I went out to the waiting area, where Misty remained seated. She said, "I'm sorry. I know he's upset about being placed. I told him I couldn't handle him." She told me she would let me know what happened. She shuffled out the main office door so she could give him a ride home.

* * *

Misty contacted me several months later and reported that Arty was doing well. "He's in a residential placement. He's completing high school. And he's in a drug program. I visit him every other week. We've been talking a lot. His mother is still at the day treatment center. I told him I was going to tell you how he was doing. He said to say hi."

I thought that would be the last time I would hear from Misty. I admired her strength and devotion. Arty had taken advantage of her; he stole money from her, abused substances, and defied her authority. I respected how she continued to be his primary support. However, agreeing to place him in a residential facility was her best choice.

Misty continued to maintain contact with me while Arty was in the placement. She finally asked to meet with me again just before Arty had completed his program. He would leave in a month, after he turned eighteen. She said she wanted my advice about a recent request he made to her. I gave her an appointment.

* * *

When I entered the waiting room, she immediately greeted me with a broad grin. I hadn't seen her in almost two years. She was seated in a motorized wheelchair and looked comfortable. I asked her to come into my office, and she adeptly navigated the vehicle, slowly maneuvering into my office and turning around so she faced my chair.

Over the years, we had developed a trusting and comfortable relationship. She had kept me informed of Arty's progress during our phone calls. She would occasionally rely on me for parenting suggestions. I knew she must have had a particular reason for wanting to meet. She was always direct and to the point, so I waited for her to let me know the purpose of her visit.

"Arty is completing his program and needs a place to live," she said. "He wants to know if he can live in my apartment."

I had always known Misty to be decisive. But clearly she was hesitant about Arty's request. She was unable to manage him before, and surely she must have been afraid it would be the same this time. She was meeting regularly with him and had to be aware of his progress. I asked what her concerns were.

"I don't know if I can manage him," she said. "I have bad memories of him living with me before. We had no trust."

I realized she was not confident that he had made significant enough progress in his treatment. She was afraid he was manipulating her for a place to live. I explained to her that, even though he was eighteen, she could still set up rules for him being in her household. She could require him to work, attend counseling, and pay for his rent and food. She listened.

"I always cared for him," she said. "I felt bad for him that he had no parent who could support him. I remember the times he would come home late at night. I would hear him come in. I knew he was up to no good—drugs, whatever other trouble. I would worry. The next day I would make sure and cook a nice meal. He would clean up and shower, and we would eat together as if nothing happened. It was our time together."

Misty grasped her wheelchair's joystick and moved the chair closer to me. She said, "I want to read something that Arty wrote to me." She pulled out a small, purple purse from the side pocket of her seat. From the purse, she pulled out a sheet of paper, unfolded it, and straightened her back. She said, "Arty told me to read you this letter. He told me to read it to you to help me decide whether he should be allowed back into my apartment." She began to read:

* * *

Dear Gammy,

This letter I am writing to you is very hard. My counselor, Mr. Freed, gave it to me to do for homework. He gives me a lot of homework. You know I am getting out of this program. I have to have a place to live. I am writing this letter to you because I realize that you care about me. All I do in this place is think. I never took this much time to think before. Mr. Freed is helping me with my thinking. I never wanted to go to counseling. I thought it was what made my mother the way she was. You always tried to make me go. I never thought I needed help. I go every week now. It helps. You were right. Mr. Freed gives me homework every week. He told me to think about my father. You were right he is a mean man. I completed a substance abuse program so I don't end up like him. I'm done with him. When I thought about my mother I realized she could hardly deal with herself and couldn't be a parent. My father and mother couldn't help me, and they made me feel angry and I didn't care. Then I thought about you. You cared. You wanted me to get help. You believed in me. I believe in me now, too. I was wrong. I did bad things. I didn't care. Drugs helped me not think, feel, or care. I don't do drugs anymore.

I completed a drug program. I completed an anger management class and got my GED. I want to make my life right. I am soon finishing this program. I need a place to live. I have to get a job.

When I went to counseling before we played Uno. I hated to be told I had to go. I learned to win with a secret stash. Ask Dr. Propp about this. Ask him if you could be my winning secret stash. Mr. Freed has been in contact with him. I signed a release.

I am writing this to you because I know you care. I am sorry for what I did. I am asking for another chance. I am a better person because I think; I think before I act. I feel I can do better and I want to do better and I am asking for your help.

Love,

Arty

Misty had a warm, pleased expression as she finished reading and folded the letter back into her purple purse. When she looked up again, she had tears in her eyes. I said, "Arty is right—you are his secret winner. You have always been there for him. I believe he has made some changes. He wants a chance to make things better."

When the session ended, she skillfully turned her wheelchair toward my office door. I opened the door for her, and she thanked me for listening to his letter. "Talk to you later," she said. "I have to work on getting Arty's room ready!"

CHALLENGES AND REFLECTIONS

The challenge in this case was how to engage a child who didn't trust adults. Arty was resistant to therapy. Arty had to accept the limitations of his parents. They were unable to care for him. He was angry at them. He resented them. He had trouble expressing this in treatment. Misty struggled to get him to come to his sessions.

Misty was devoted to Arty's care. She had seen genuine qualities in him. She realized how incapable his parents were. As a teenager Arty showed a lack of respect for Misty. He engaged in risky, delinquent actions. He took advantage of her.

Arty became unmanageable. He had to be placed in a secure environment.

In the residential facility, Arty had mandatory counseling. He benefited from this treatment. He learned that he reacted and had not thought about his actions. He began to understand how much Misty meant to him. She was the only one to regularly visit him. She continued to believe in him. Misty acknowledged her commitment to Arty in a parent session. She would often come in alone to talk about Arty. She cared for him. She wanted to give him another chance. After Arty's release, she would allow him to move back in with her.

Chapter 8

Sam and Shira

PRESENTING PROBLEMS

Sam (seven) and Shira (six) were brought into treatment by their mother Emily. Her therapist recommended the children be seen. This was after Emily received a report from their teachers about their recent problematic behaviors in school. Emily was a single parent. She was devoted to her children. She was careful about her relationships with men. This wasn't how she was raised by her mother.

She made a parenting decision that affected her children. She chose a sitter to watch them one evening. She started dating a man. It was not well thought out. The person taking care of them engaged Sam and Shira in inappropriate activities. After the incident, the children acted differently.

In this case, Ruth saw Shira, while I saw Sam. We assessed Sam and Shira. We found out they were acting differently because of the sitter incident. The children each shared their version of what had happened. In family therapy, we helped the children explain to Emily the manipulative event. We made a mandated report together with Emily.

TREATMENT STORY

Emily had clearly had an unhappy childhood. She never knew her father, and her mother resented being a parent. She was rarely home. Emily had many different caregivers, but she didn't remember anyone special. When her mother was home, she was often angry, and she said nasty things about Emily's father. Eventually Emily stopped asking about him.

Now Emily was a mother. Her children, Sam and Shira, had different fathers. She was not aware of where Shira's father was, but Matt, Sam's father, was helpful and reliably took both children for his scheduled visitation every other weekend. He helped with child support. Emily had respect for Matt and believed he was a good father.

The kids had never met their grandmother, and Emily had not spoken to her in years. If they even thought of the fact that their mother must have parents of her own, they never mentioned it. Like her own mother, Emily was a single parent. She found it difficult, and she was often overwhelmed. But unlike her mother, Emily worked hard at being a good parent. She attended therapy, and over time, she gained an understanding of her mother's poor parenting. She wanted to raise her children differently. She had strong instincts and a good heart, but her childhood experience of dysfunctional parenting often crossed her up.

Those conflicting attributes came to a head when she went to her children's school for teacher conferences.

Sam was seven years old and in first grade. His teacher told Emily that he had changed recently. Usually a conscientious student, he had stopped doing his classwork a couple of weeks ago. He'd been surly with his teacher and told her that he didn't care about school. This new attitude was startling.

Something similar was going on with Shira, who was six years old and in kindergarten. Like Sam, she had stopped participating. She had always been responsible and eager in class, but now she just sulked at her table. Shira's teacher asked if anything had happened at home.

The question sent a chill down Emily's spine. Yes, she believed something may have happened at home. She had already suspected as much. She just didn't know what. She discussed it with her therapist, who suggested that the children should see a counselor. That's when Emily contacted us about seeing Sam and Shira.

* * *

Before having the children in for sessions, Ruth met with Emily to review the family history. Emily told Ruth about her childhood with her mother and her life as a single parent. She felt guilty because sometimes she was so exhausted after work she didn't take the time to ask her kids about their school day. She worried that she had neglected them like her mother did to her. She went on to describe some of the changes she was trying to make in order to be a better parent. After their meeting, Ruth caught me up on this history.

"Trusting men isn't one of Emily's strengths," Ruth told me as we sat in her office. I listened while sitting on her smaller two-person couch and looking at the drawings on her corkboard. The pictures were of landscapes, scenes, and anime characters. Ruth warned me that, because of Emily's issues with men, she might not warm to me at first. "She confessed to having a number of unsuccessful relationships with men. None of these interactions resulted in a stable long-term partner. Recently she's been trying to be more careful about the men she has in her home. Her mother always had her boyfriends over. One of the men made her feel very uncomfortable when she was about Shira's age. She's been working with her therapist on this."

Ruth believed that Emily had gained a lot from her own therapy. She had changed her actions toward men and had learned to be more cautious. Emily proudly told Ruth that she had recently been promoted to management at her job with the Main Street Food Supply Company. Besides the obvious benefit of higher pay, her new position came with a work schedule that allowed her to be more available to her kids and keep them in day care less.

Since starting her treatment, Emily had not dated except for one brief relationship. She told Ruth she recently ended this relationship.

The man's name was Paul.

She first met him several months ago, when he was working part time in maintenance at her facility. They would talk almost every day at lunch. After he left for another job, he started messaging her, asking if she wanted to date. She talked to her therapist about the man. She liked him but wasn't sure if she was ready to be involved. In the past, she'd met men at parties or on a dating website, but this was different. She wanted to be a better parent now. The pact she made with herself and her therapist was to go slow and not introduce a man to her children until she had made a significant commitment to him.

She began to see Paul during the weekends when the kids were at Matt's house. After dating for a while, Paul asked her if she would like to come over to his apartment. They were becoming more physically intimate. In past relationships, sex had always come first. She had waited this time and felt she might be ready.

On the night of their date, however, her babysitter became ill and canceled on her. The children were not with Matt that weekend. Paul suggested that his roommate Nick could watch the children. The kids had met him before, when Emily and the kids ran into him and Paul in the grocery store. Emily had a feeling that this might not be the best situation, but without thinking it through carefully, she agreed. Nick seemed like a nice man. He reminded her of a big kid. He told her he would play games with them.

That night, the men came over to her apartment. The children seemed fine with Nick staying with them. She expected to return to the apartment early in the evening after they were asleep.

"As she described the evening," Ruth told me, "she seemed to get upset. She had difficulty talking about it. She eventually told me what occurred."

It was Emily's first time at Paul's apartment. The place seemed messy to her, but she thought that's the way men live. They had drinks and talked. After a while, Paul asked her to watch a porn film, and then maybe try what they saw. This was unnerving enough to Emily, but then he told her the sex movies belonged to his roommate. As Emily looked through the names of the films, she told Ruth, "I started to have a bad feeling in my stomach." One of the titles was something about young school girls.

Seeing that, Emily began to have doubts about Nick being with her children. She told Paul she wanted to leave right away. She felt queasy about viewing Nick's pornography with him, and she told Paul she was feeling sick and nauseous. He became upset and concerned and pleaded with her not to go home, but reluctantly he drove her back to her apartment. They parted ways amicably, and he waited in his car for Nick. When Emily entered her place, the children were sleeping. She asked Nick how everything went, and he told her everything was just fine. "Nothing to worry about," he told her. He said they played a game and had fun.

Ruth asked Emily if she noticed any difference in how the children acted after that evening. Emily told her that the next evening she found the children playing in their pajamas in Shira's closet. When she asked them what they were doing, they said they were playing a game Uncle Nick taught them.

"The 'Uncle Nick' name was disturbing to Emily," Ruth said, shutting her notebook and setting it on her desk. "The whole thing about Paul wanting her to watch porn, Nick being alone with her kids, hiding in the closet—and now she finds out he was saying he was their uncle—the whole thing made her feel very uneasy."

Emily told her therapist about the uneasy feelings and the fact that the situation brought up some scary childhood memories for her. Her therapist supported her in her wish to end the relationship with Paul. She contacted him and said it was over. Her therapist said she had concerns about Nick as well.

We were now prepared to meet with the children. We believed that the evening Nick watched them might have had something to do with both children's behavior changes. We scheduled an appointment with Emily to bring Sam and Shira in.

* * *

Ruth and I came out to the waiting room to meet the three of them. Emily, a petite, pretty woman, immediately looked at Ruth. Ruth smiled at her and said, "This is my co-therapist, Dr. Propp. He will be seeing Sam." Sam sat on her left and Shira on her right. Both had dark hair and were of short stature like their mother. Emily only quickly glanced at me, but Sam made eye contact. I said to him, "Would you like to play with the toys in my office?"

Ruth reminded Emily that she would be seeing Shira while I was with Sam. Ruth then reassured her, "After our meetings with the children, we will all meet together to talk about what was shared."

Sam stood up and followed my lead into my office. I directed him to the multipurpose children's table. I had previously taken the cover off so I could do sand play with today's patients. I said, "Your mother said Nick watched you a couple of weeks ago. She was upset about the evening and said he played an inappropriate game with you and Shira." I wanted to get right to the point and then give him some time to think about what I said. "Would you like to play with the animals in the sand?"

Sam seemed eager to respond to what I said, but he wanted to play, too. He said, "What animals?"

I took the bins of wild animals and dinosaurs off the shelf and opened them up. I placed the bins next to him on the floor. "Here are the animals," I said.

He began to put some of the animals in the sand, and attending to the animals seemed to comfort him.

I asked, "What happened with Nick?"

"He started showing us this YouTube video and said we would play the game," he said. "This Foxy character jumped out, and I told him I didn't want to watch anymore. Shira didn't like it either—she wouldn't even look at the video."

"Did he listen to you?" I asked. He stopped playing with animals and looked at me. He seemed fearful about what he was going to say.

"He did, but then he said, 'let's play the game.' He would be a security guard and we had to hide. Then he would try and find us."

I wondered what frightened him. "Was something scary about the Foxy character in the video?"

"He had a patch over his eye and a hook for a hand. And it felt like he jumped at me," he said. "I keep dreaming about him."

"The video was only a made-up story and not real," I said. "Let's make up our own story with the animals."

He grabbed a tiger and a dinosaur and started to move them to different areas in the sand. I said, "Maybe the dinosaur can guard the tiger. Can you make a story about them?"

Sam said, "This dinosaur is guarding the tiger. The tiger is hiding and jumps out and scares the dinosaur. But the dinosaur stops him." He hid the tiger behind a pile of sand.

"That was a great story, kind of like the YouTube video Nick showed you. You made it up and it's only a story," I said. "Like the Foxy character who is not real."

Sam became more relaxed, and his fearful look faded. He asked if he could play with the farm.

While he was setting up the farm and barn animals, I asked him more direct questions about Nick.

He said, "I don't like Nick." I asked why, and he said, "He tried to grab me in the game."

"Did he touch you?" I asked.

He said, "No way! I told my mom I never want to see him again." He moved a horse through the sand for a moment, then he added, "I know he's not my uncle."

I believed Sam was clear and up-front about the details of what happened the evening Nick watched them. He had good instincts and judgment. Even so, I was concerned because Nick engaged the children in inappropriate game play and crossed boundaries. While Sam played with the farm, I checked with Ruth by speakerphone about her session with Shira. This was in preparation for our meeting with Emily.

Ruth told me that Shira played out the evening's event using the dollhouse. She had a doll for a security guard and two little dolls representing children.

The story she described was similar to the one Sam told me.

Ruth said, "Shira has a good understanding of safety and reported no inappropriate touching. She does not want to see Nick again. After processing the event, Shira seemed less impacted." Ruth agreed with me that Nick crossed boundaries in his play behavior with the children and their mother needed to be informed.

Ruth brought Shira into my office. Sam and I put away the farm, and Ruth began playing a card game with them while I went to get their mother so we could all meet.

I prepared Emily as we walked together to my office. I informed her that we were troubled by Nick's behavior. We believed his actions affected the children and contributed to the difficulties they were having. When Emily and I entered the room, the children stopped playing. She sat on the couch, and the children sat on each side of her.

Ruth helped Shira explain what she shared in her therapy. Quite excited to speak first, as evidenced by her facial expression and the sparkle in her large brown eyes, she shared what she understood from her talk.

"We talked about my body, and how it is *my* body." Then she said, "We can say, *No!*"

"That is a powerful statement," Ruth said. "Can you tell your mother more of what saying the word *No* means?"

"It's my body," she said.

"What does that mean about touch?" Ruth asked.

"If I don't want anyone to touch me," Shira continued, "I can say no, because it's my body."

Emily's face beamed, and her brown eyes welled up as she listened to her daughter's assertive words. Sam, too, spoke of how he controlled his body. Emily observed her children's empowerment as they asserted they had the right to give consent to anyone who wanted to touch their bodies.

We wanted Emily to understand that the children had a good sense of sexual boundaries. They each reacted immediately when Nick attempted to touch them.

Emily said, "He tried to touch them!"

"He did," Ruth said, "but they resisted and knew what to do."

"I never talked to them about having appropriate boundaries with adults. How did they know what to do?" Emily asked.

"Shira and Sam have good instincts," Ruth said. "You can always support their intuitive sense with some appropriate reading material."

Emily appeared interested. I handed her a list of books that the local library had available for parents. I placed marks next to the books for her to read with them first. Sam asked, "Could we go to the library?" Emily agreed.

Next, we helped the children describe to Emily what happened that evening with Nick. I asked Sam to begin and talk about the game they played.

Sam said, "Uncle Nick put on this video—"

Emily's mouth dropped. "I told you not to call him that."

"Sorry," Sam replied. "I forgot." He looked at me. "He said to call him Uncle Nick. He said it would be our secret."

Quite visibly upset, Emily blurted out, "You don't have an Uncle Nick. That man is not your uncle!"

Sam looked at the floor in deference to his mother. I discussed how adults attempt to gain children's trust by telling them they were closer than they really were and telling them secrets, like calling themselves a relative such as an uncle when they were not, and telling a child something was a secret when it really was not.

Ruth said, "If he was your uncle, your mother would have told you." Emily nodded in agreement.

"People you don't know shouldn't tell you secrets," Ruth added.

To this, their mother said, "I'm sorry. I should have never let Nick watch you." She rubbed the bridge of her nose and looked down into her lap.

"Be careful about secrets. Nick told you to keep secrets. You have been honest with your mother. Keeping secrets from her didn't make you feel good."

I commented that adults can make you feel uneasy when they invade your personal space or "bubble." Both children said, "Yes!"

"Nick wasn't nice to you," I went on. "He told you to keep secrets from your mother. That's not okay. Nick said he was your uncle when he wasn't, and he wanted you to play a game that was not for children your age. That was not being sensitive to your needs, and it was not making you feel safe."

Emily finally looked at me directly and appeared to be pleased with what I said.

I asked Sam to explain more about the game they played.

"He showed the game on YouTube. I didn't like it. This Foxy guy jumps out and scares you."

Shira contorted her face and said, "I closed my eyes."

Sam continued, "Nick told us he would be the security guard. We would have to hide from him."

"Do you remember what you told me you didn't like?" I asked Sam.

He responded with hesitancy in his voice. "He wanted us to take off our clothes and hide. I didn't want to. He said it's how you play the game."

Shira immediately became upset and looked at her mother. "I told him you told me never to undress in front of strangers."

I encouraged Sam to tell his mother what he had told me. "We said we would play the game, but in our jammies," the boy said.

"It was what we sleep in anyway," Shira said.

I added that the children told us they changed in their own rooms. Nick wanted to come in, but they said no to him.

At this point, Emily had balled up her fist and pressed it into her lap, visibly agitated and angry. "I should have never let Nick in my apartment. I came home early because I had a bad feeling about him. I'm so sorry," she said, shaking her head. "I should have been a better mother."

To help her see the positive aspect of her parenting, I said, "Sam and Shira did a great job at protecting themselves. Nick made them uncomfortable. He had limited regard for them as children and made them feel unsafe. The idea of playing a game was intriguing, and sparked their interest, but nevertheless the children held their ground. They demonstrated a good sense of right and wrong behaviors. That was because of your parenting."

Sam talked more about the game. "He told us to hide in the closet. It was like hide and seek. We hid in our jammies."

"Tell your mother what you said to me about the game," Ruth said to Shira.

"I didn't like it," Shira said. "He turned the lights off."

"Then," Sam added, "he made noises. He kept saying, '*Where are you?*' He said he was going to get us."

"We held each other," Shira said. "Uncle Nick—I'm sorry, Mommy, I mean Nick—said he was the security guard. He opened the door."

"How did you feel at that moment?" Ruth asked.

"I was really scared and held Sam so tight. When he came in I screamed, and when he tried to grab us, I yelled, *I don't want to play!*"

"What did you do then?" I asked as I looked at Sam.

"We ran out," Sam said. "We told him we don't want to play anymore. We told him we wanted to go to bed."

According to what we gathered, at that point Nick told them to go to bed and to keep the game as their little secret. We thanked Sam and Shira for helping their mother understand what happened. We said they did a great job in saying no to Nick. The children said they were relieved after explaining the entire incident to their mother.

We wanted to have a follow-up meeting with Emily alone as soon as possible. We felt the incident with Nick needed further attention. Emily agreed, and we were able to coordinate a time for an appointment early the following week.

* * *

I started the session. This time, Emily was able to look at me directly. I believed she had more trust in what I had to say. I said, "Ruth and I have some serious concerns about Nick's behavior with Shira and Sam. How did you feel after hearing them talk about the evening?"

Emily took a deep breath as if to gather her thoughts. It was clear she had taken some time to sort through the incident. But although she seemed collected, there was fury in her voice as she said, "I hate that man. He wanted my children to take off their clothes. He wanted to touch them. He is sick. I wish I could have him arrested."

Ruth tried to comfort her. "Shira and Sam are wonderful children. We enjoyed them. They handled the situation well."

"I saw my therapist yesterday," Emily said. "She helped me understand why I became so upset. It might have to do with my own abuse. I was feeling so bad for trusting Nick with my children. I was feeling like I did something very wrong—like I was a bad parent."

"We all can make mistakes," I said. "Shira and Sam talked honestly about what happened, and you supported their decisions."

"Over the weekend, we spent some family time together watching a movie and playing some games," Emily replied. "It felt special."

I realized that Emily still felt the situation was not resolved. She continued to feel this angst that she allowed Nick to be around her children. "You seem to be still concerned about what happened," I observed.

"I have this sick feeling in my stomach when I think about Nick. My therapist said he is a trigger to what happened to me when I was around Shira's age. I should have trusted what I felt. I wanted to see Paul and maybe be with a man again. I didn't take time to think through everything. I *worried* Nick might be the kind of man that could take advantage of others. I realize now I actually did feel that. But I put it out of my mind." Emily was crying.

I grabbed a box of tissues and handed it to her. She took the box and pulled a tissue out.

"But the whole situation still doesn't feel right to me!" she said. "I broke it off with Paul. I got the kids help. But I still don't feel okay about it."

Ruth and I looked at each other. We both knew how we were going to respond. Ruth said, "We would like to report the incident. Nick's behavior with the children was sexually inappropriate. He also seems to be in possession of child pornography." Emily looked up after dabbing her eyes. She seemed receptive. I explained that, even though the children were currently safe from the man, we believed that his actions were serious enough to report. We planned to contact Child Protective Services by phone. We wanted her to participate in the call.

"What do you mean?" she asked.

Ruth explained, "The hotline is a twenty-four-hour service to report suspected child abuse or neglect. We would like to call while you are here with us. This would allow you to give specific details. You would be better able to describe the pornography DVDs you saw."

I said that we will explain what the children told us in therapy about Nick's exploitive behavior. We will discuss how Nick enticed them to engage in an inappropriate game in which he attempted to touch them. I conveyed to her that it was our hope that the content of the incident, and the possession of child pornography, would encourage the police to at least investigate Nick.

Emily appeared pleased and said, "I would feel better if Nick could be checked out by the police. I hope he gets what he deserves."

She consented to our plan. I placed the phone on speaker and dialed the number. The intake social worker on the line introduced herself. I explained we wanted to report an abuse incident involving two young children. The worker immediately asked if the children were currently safe. We assured her they are. She requested basic demographics first, as well as descriptions of the incident.

Emily sat straight up, looked at the phone, and presented her information. She gave the address of the apartment, the complete names of the men, and the names of the movies she saw. We discussed how the man was intrusive and attempted to groom the children to engage in inappropriate sexualized activities. He said he was their uncle, he told them to keep what happened a secret, and he attempted to touch them.

When the call was completed, Emily let out another deep breath and smiled at us. She appeared relieved. We advocated for informing Sam's father about the situation, and Emily agreed. "I want to tell him." If he needed to meet with us, he had the right as part of the custody arrangement, I reminded her.

* * *

Emily, Shira, and Sam continued to come in for regular sessions after that. I met with Sam, and he would happily play at the sand table with different figures and toy items. He eventually stopped thinking about Foxy and never brought up Nick again. Ruth met with Shira at the same time. Every meeting ended with a family session. Ruth and I made an effort to help support Emily's parenting decisions. She was clear and consistent about the household rules and set up fair consequences.

Over time, Emily let go of her anger and frustrations with herself for inviting Nick into her household. The five of us were sitting in my office for a family session when Emily said, "I feel so much better as a mother. I had all these doubts and worries, you know? I've had to learn how to be a good mother. But the more I listen to and understand my children, the better I do."

"Yeah, we can tell Mom everything," Shira added.

Emily met with the kids' teachers, who reported that both Sam and Shira were buckling down in class again. The children continued to develop a strong bond with their mother, and she made an effort to reflect on each day's events when they were together as a family in the evening.

"I've been reading them the books you recommended," Emily said. "It's helped us feel closer as a family."

Emily used in her home the organizational skills she demonstrated at work that had resulted in her promotion. She established a weekly meal plan and had each child choose their favorite dinner once a week. She developed household rules: She set up chores for each of them, scheduled homework time, and had them follow consistent bedtimes. In addition, she limited Shira's and Sam's screen time, and she monitored what games they played and the content of the material they watched.

"I always wanted to be a good mother," Emily concluded, "but I didn't think I knew how. All I knew was that it wasn't how I was brought up. My mother never talked to me or listened to me. I thought she didn't care. We had no rules. But then I realized I needed to trust myself and believe that I am a good mother and I am not like my mother was."

Emily, at one point, informed us that the children had been interviewed by Child Protective Services. Nick was being investigated.

As our time with the family ended, Emily shared with us privately that Nick was charged with the possession of child pornography.

CHALLENGES AND REFLECTIONS

Emily worked hard at being a competent single parent. She was adamant about not repeating her own problematic upbringing. Her mother was neglectful; she was interested in men and not her daughter. Emily understood the importance of paying attention to her children's needs. She wanted them to feel safe.

As a child therapist, I know it is important to develop a relationship with the caregiver. My challenge was to acknowledge Emily's mistrust of men. I followed Ruth's lead. I was careful in how I spoke to Emily. I was sensitive to her and tried not to be pushy.

Emily wanted to understand why her children were behaving differently. She had good instincts about parenting. She needed validation and support. She felt sad and hurt because of her poor parenting decision.

Ruth gathered that Emily was probably victimized as a child. Ruth understood this from the way she talked about her own childhood. Emily as a parent had a heathy relationship with her children. This made Ruth believe that Emily was dealing with these problems in her therapy.

As co-therapists, Ruth and I knew we had to make a report about the baby-sitter's actions with Sam and Shira. We agreed that it was important to include Emily in making this mandated report. We all made the call together. This seemed to help Emily feel empowered. She believed she was doing the right thing. She wanted to identify the man who took advantage of her children.

Chapter 9

Is Doug Disabled?

PRESENTING PROBLEMS

Doug was a seven-year-old boy. His mother, Joan, brought him in for therapy. This was a first for Joan; she had never been to a therapist before. I didn't understand her reasons for having Doug in treatment. I thought she wanted him to get on disability like his older brothers. This would be a help to the family financially. Then I realized that she thought I could get him to go to school.

Doug's mother had limited finances and lived in a subsidized apartment. Jeff, their father, lived off the land in a crudely built cabin. Joan sincerely wanted to do the best she could for Doug. She saw that he was different from his older brothers. They were both disabled. As I engaged Doug in therapy, I realized that he was unique. His play interactions were creative and unusual.

I didn't expect Doug to remain in therapy. But he welcomed the therapeutic process. He continued to work with me until his teenage years. He was motivated to be the first in his family to complete high school. Doug cleverly figured out his way of breaking the cycle of poverty by developing his own business.

TREATMENT STORY

It was one of those fall mornings that I decided to take the back way into the office. I left the house slightly later, so I would miss the school buses. On the ride, I enjoyed my time looking at the red, yellow, and orange colors of the maple leaves. I heard the sound of tractors grinding as the area farmers were harvesting the fields. When I got into my office, I took off my light jacket and listened to my voice messages. I heard, "This is Joan! Doug won't get up and go to school!" I thought maybe Joan had mistakenly called my office instead of the school. But I returned her call. When Joan answered, I asked if she had contacted me looking for a child therapist.

She hesitated. "Yeah? I can't get Doug to go to school. I never had this problem with his older brothers."

I decided that it might be better if I talked to her in person so I could understand the concerns in more detail. I suggested she and the boy's father come in for the first appointment.

"Big Jeff doesn't live with us, and he won't come," she said. "Should I bring Doug?"

I said I would like to meet with her alone first before I had a session with her son.

* * *

Joan arrived promptly and remained seated in the far corner of the waiting room by the entrance. She resisted making eye contact when I looked in her direction. I noticed her plaid shirt, dark cargo pants, and old pair of boots. Her shoddy dress confirmed what I suspected from our cryptic phone conversation. She was culturally limited and wouldn't usually be inclined to use our services. I introduced myself and asked her to come with me into my office.

She sat down on the couch and said, "Can you get him to go to school?"

I could tell she had not been to a therapist before. It almost felt like she expected me to take Doug to school. But I assumed she genuinely felt challenged by her son's behavior and wanted some help. I handed her the intake forms and pointed out to her where to sign the consent to treatment so we could discuss her son. She started to slowly print her name in large capital letters. I said, "You can just sign your name and I will fill out the paperwork while we talk."

She said, "I need help with Doug."

"How did you hear about me?" I wondered.

"You helped my sister, Brianna, with her daughter, Sophia," she said.

Ethically I couldn't say whether or not I had seen her sister. But I remembered Brianna and Sophia and saw some physical similarities she had with her sister. Brianna was developmentally disabled, and when I evaluated Sophia, who was about three at the time, she seemed to be quite intellectually limited as well. After I saw them, I immediately referred them to the local mental health center for services. I set up an appointment for them while they were in my office. Brianna had no understanding what to do for her child and was especially appreciative of the help, I recalled.

I said, "I would like to learn more about Doug from you. But first, let's start with everyone's age in the family."

She told me Doug was seven. I was surprised when she told me she was thirty-eight. She appeared to be twenty years older than that. She said she resided in a rent-subsidized apartment with Doug and her two older boys. She had dropped out of school and never worked. She appeared to not be as developmentally impaired as I remembered her sister Brianna to be. She said she wasn't on disability.

"My older boys are on disability, and neither of them made it through school," she said.

I wondered if she was seeking disability benefits for Doug. This type of benefit provides more income for a family. Was Doug disabled?

Joan believed that he was not like his older brothers.

"I think Doug is smarter than the others. He likes to learn things," she told me. "When I show him how to do something, he does it right. His brothers, I have to tell them over and over. They forget. Doug, he remembers. I bet he'll be the first in the family to finish school. Me and his father never did."

Her oldest son was Jeff, who was eighteen. From the description she shared, he appeared to be socially isolated. "He stays in his room playing video games. He don't have no friends. I can't get him to leave. He won't walk to the store with us."

Her middle child, Wayne, was sixteen. About him, she said, "His teachers said he couldn't learn. He sat in class. He never did no work. I didn't bother to send him anymore."

"What about the boys' father?" I asked. "Why doesn't he live with you?"

"Big Jeff!" she said. "We never married. Big Jeff sees the boys. When he wants to. He lives off the land. He has a cabin in the woods. He does logging." As she presented the information about the boys' father, her smile left me with a feeling that she admired the man.

I inquired about her and Big Jeff's respective family histories. She shared that there were no substance abuse problems in her family background. It sounded like her parents were extremely poor. They rented a trailer in one of the most rundown parks in the area. Her sister lived with them. She admitted that Big Jeff drank and had a history of alcohol abuse and mental illness in his family. "He can't read or write. I help him do his bills. I tell him how much wood he needs to sell," she explained.

I was curious if Big Jeff would be willing to come in to discuss the children. I thought, since he spends some time with the boys, maybe he could share his perspective. I always like to get input from both parents.

She instantly stated, "No! He won't talk, especially to no counselor."

In reviewing Doug's early childhood, Joan remembered a serious medical incident that had occurred when he was three years old. She recalled he had had a severe hand injury that resulted in him having two bent fingers on his left hand.

Joan reflected, "It was when we lived at Big Jeff's. That's when the state made us leave his place."

As she recalled the event in a somewhat disjointed manner, I gathered the following: Doug was with his father in the woods. They came back to the cabin with his left hand wrapped in his father's shirt and blood all over the place. She said something about the shirt smelling of alcohol. I asked if she thought Jeff might have been drinking. She responded, "Big Jeff said he poured moonshine on it." I left it at that, even though I had concerns that he might have been drinking and might have been more a part of the accident than she was aware.

She continued, "I remember Doug screaming in pain." I asked her if she had any idea how the injury might have happened.

She said, "Big Jeff never says much. He said Doug fell. He fell on the chain saw, he said." She told me the blood frightened her. She drove him to the hospital with Wayne's help. Once at the emergency room, she explained, his hand was placed in some kind of bandage where his fingers were attached together.

"Doug didn't like that bandage," she said sadly. "He ripped it off. The doctors messed up. His fingers are bent to this day." She said that they had to move out of Big Jeff's self-built cabin after that.

I asked, "What happened?"

"Doug said his father did it," Joan said. So a state caseworker made a home safety inspection and determined that the place wasn't safe for children. "The stuff she said in court," Joan recalled, "like no running water, the woodstove was not okay, and wires were all over the floor. Well, Big Jeff got water from the stream. He cut his own wood for heat. The place was warm. I don't get why they made us move."

I gathered that Big Jeff managed to live cheaply off the grid. She also stated he was a "good provider."

"We always had food," she said. "He's a bow hunter. He butchers the meat himself." She chuckled and added, "At least when they came to the cabin, they didn't find the moonshine. Or the weed he grows."

The state caseworker was helpful and assisted them with obtaining the rent-subsidized apartment they currently lived in.

Finally feeling comfortable after telling her family's story, she agreed to bring Doug in so I could meet with him.

"What do I do if he don't go to school?" she asked.

My advice to her was not to pressure him. Let me see if I could figure out what the problem might be when I saw him the next week.

* * *

The following week, Doug and his mother were in the waiting room. Joan sat in the same chair wearing her boots again and, I thought, maybe the same outfit she had on when she saw me the previous week. Doug had on an old pair of jeans that looked loose and well worn, as if they'd been handed down by his older brother. He sat at the children's table playing with the blocks, though he was a big kid and dwarfed the table. He looked right at me when I came out to get him and seemed excited for our meeting. His mother introduced me as "the doctor that don't give needles."

I showed Doug my office. He eyed the space, looking first at the bins of toys on the shelf. He then pointed to the drawings that other children had done and were displayed on the large corkboard. "I like those," he said.

"Would you like to choose some toys to play with?" I asked. I was intrigued by his interest and curiosity, and already I was concluding that he probably wasn't limited.

He gravitated to the bin containing the rubber wild animals. We talked about the different kinds of wild animals. I proposed we open up the sand table and arrange the toy figures according to animal families. He liked the idea, and we placed ourselves at the table.

"Let's make homes for the beasts," he said.

I was impressed that he took control of the play activity. I grabbed a box of wooden blocks and put them next to him.

I observed him as he meticulously separated out and defined living spaces. He used the wooden blocks to construct the structures. "This is where the water animals will go, the lions and tigers I can put in the corner, and I'm making a special place for the baby animals," he explained.

Doug was organized and bright. He allowed himself to become absorbed and soothed through the meditative quality of his play. As he began to appear relaxed, I asked him why he didn't want to go to school. I gave him some time to respond to my question. I didn't want to interrupt his play. After a while he said, "The teacher doesn't like me. I don't have any friends. Why do I have to go?"

I said to him, "School is important for you to learn things. Your mother told me she was concerned, because some mornings you refused to go to school. She told me she didn't know why you didn't want to go."

He complained, "I'm tired. I can't sleep. I don't like going when I'm tired."

I asked, "Do you have trouble sleeping at night?"

"Yeah, I do. But I stay up and play video games," he said.

I said, "Sleep is important. I could see why you wouldn't want to go to school if you were tired."

He thought about what I said and, interestingly, responded with, "Even the beasts of the jungle sleep."

I wondered how much he understood sleep. "Where would the animals sleep?" I asked, pointing to the animal families he had carefully laid out in the sand box. He proceeded to add flat wooden blocks to the animal areas he had developed.

He stated, "Now the beasts have beds. They have a place to sleep."

I stated that sleep helped animals have strength to hunt for food. I commented that children, when they slept well, would be more alert for the next school day.

When it was time for his mother to be part of the treatment, we planned what we would talk about with her. He said I could discuss his sleep issues and school concerns.

I shared with Joan that Doug told me he didn't sleep well on some nights. He said he didn't like going to school when he was tired. I proposed that we come up with a sleep plan. Doug listened intently as he continued his play. His mother admitted to not having a sleep routine or clear bedtime, and she consented to introducing a nighttime plan. The plan I suggested included setting an appropriate bedtime for his age and nighttime rules. I said there should be no video or game screens an hour before bed. I looked at Doug and said he could read a story or listen to music instead. I smiled and reminded him not to forget to brush his teeth every night.

He expressed his interest with a head nod and said, "I like it. I'll try it."

As our time ended, I again reviewed the sleep hygiene plan with Doug and his mother. I assisted him with putting away the toys. He talked about playing with the animals again when he returned.

* * *

Over the next few months, Doug had several sessions. He managed over time to develop better sleeping habits, and his school attendance improved. I had explained to Joan that Doug was different from his older brothers. He was not disabled. He liked coming to his sessions.

Near the end of the school year, I negotiated a plan to meet with them over the summer. We would have three visits: one in July, one in August, and one the week before school. I thought summer would be a beneficial time to assess Doug without the stress of him having to go to school.

However, Doug missed the July visit. His mother called at a later time. I gently let her know that it was important to at least contact me, rather than not show up. I wanted to help her understand that she needs to cancel the session beforehand.

She committed to bringing Doug into an appointment before the start of school. When Doug came in, he immediately engaged with the animals at the sand table. But his play had a different quality. It was more disorganized and aggressive. He just took out the rubber wild animals and had them fight each other in the sand box.

I asked him, "What did you do over the summer?"

He said, "I stayed up all night. I played on the Play Station. I don't like going out. There's nothing to do. The kids fight on the playground. Teenagers pick on us."

Doug seemed very tired, but I managed to help him arrange the animals into families like he did before. I had his mother come in.

Joan told me that she conformed to the summer culture of the housing project. Most people were up at night and slept late into the day. She said, "It's cooler at night. We can't have no air conditioners. We only have fans."

I realized Doug's sleep schedule had become reversed. I knew I had to introduce some kind of sleep strategy to get him ready for school, so I devised a plan. I encouraged the boy to remain awake the entire night on Saturday. School would start three days later. But, I said, the challenge was that he would have to not fall asleep the next day until his normal school bedtime. This would help reset his sleep schedule.

He and his mother were intrigued by the plan. His mother offered a way to help keep him awake: "I'll take Wayne and him swimming. We can stay all day. He likes going. Jeff won't come."

"It can be the last of my all-nighters," Doug said.

I instructed his mother in the use of a low dose of melatonin as a sleep aid. I told her where to get some at the local pharmacy. She agreed to introduce this natural treatment an hour before his recommended bedtime after the "all-nighter." They left the session with a plan.

* * *

At our scheduled session for the second week of school, I wanted to reassess Doug's progress. He was quite comfortable coming into my office. He took out his favorite animals and set up the families as he had done in the past.

He created a special hiding place made out of blocks. "This is for the baby animals," he said. Then he built an arena out of the blocks and said, "This is where the older tigers can battle." He had the tigers attack and clash against each other, and quickly the fighting began to take on a loud, frenzied tone. I realized I needed to shift the play dynamic, so I engaged in the play scene with an alternative theme. I moved the large tiger toward where the baby animals were. I said this mother tiger was going to teach the baby tigers survival skills instead of fighting.

He liked the concept. He grabbed a large lion and did a jumping move with the little baby lion watching. He had the baby imitate the action. In this way, he changed his play from aggressive to a more cooperative and mentoring activity. The different large animals cleverly showed the smaller figures jumps, climbs, twists, and other movements, as we both manipulated them. We laughed at our demonstrations.

I asked him about his school attendance. Was he tired in the morning? I was hoping he had been following the night routine.

He said, "I sleep better. The night plan works." He manipulated the toy figures and said, "Look how this father lion trains the baby lion." He had the adult lion do a flip high above the table, followed by the baby lion doing the same.

"How's it going at school?" I asked. I had gathered from our interactions that he was a bright child. I wondered if he applied himself at school.

"I don't like it," he said sadly. "The kids are mean. They call me 'Crooked Fingers.'"

He refocused on his play. He rearranged the animals and decided to have the two strongest lions teach the babies together. He said, "The strongest animals have to teach the little ones how to protect themselves."

I went out to get his mother. I wanted to talk to her about his school difficulties and peer problems. She related how the boy's sleep had improved.

She said, "He goes every morning."

Still engaged in his play, he chimed in, "I don't like my teacher. The kids are mean." In a sad and dejected manner, he told his mother what the other students called him.

I observed his mother's caring glance. She understood he was being picked on, but I don't believe she knew how to help him. I wondered if Doug's teacher was aware of the problem. Maybe she could help. I asked Joan if she could connect with her.

She said, "I know her. I see her at the end of the day. When I pick Doug up. What should I tell her?"

I realized she might not be able to fully explain the concerns to Doug's teacher, but I wanted to give her the chance. I helped her rehearse what to say. I also said that, if this continued, I could contact his teacher as well.

* * *

After canceling several sessions in a row, Joan called to explain that Doug had been really ill. This was in the late fall. The boy came in for his next session with dark circles under his eyes, and he said, "I haven't been sleeping." He said he just returned to school after missing almost a month. He was lethargic and listlessly pulled the bin of his favorite animals off of the toy shelf. With his head in the crease of his elbow, he slowly moved the beasts around. Almost nonverbal, he remained fixated on his play.

When his mother came into my office, she appeared upset. She said she had tried to talk to his teacher like I had suggested, but the teacher didn't listen. "He doesn't like school; the kids won't leave him alone," she said.

I said, "A month is a lot of school to miss."

She complained, "The school reported Doug. They said he was truant. Now we have court. I'm afraid they'll take him from me."

I helped her understand that she probably needed a medical excuse from his doctor if Doug was so ill that he missed a month of school. She signed a release so I could talk with the assigned state caseworker. I informed her about confidentiality, assuring her that I would only discuss information she gave me permission to talk about. I said that I wanted to explain to his case-worker that Doug was being bullied and had sleep problems. I was able to ease some of her fears and worries about Doug being taken away.

Joan found the caseworker to be helpful and supportive. Next time I saw her, she told me, "She helped us get winter stuff. She got him a jacket and boots. She came over. She even took him to school."

The caseworker convened a school meeting and helped develop a plan. Doug would meet regularly with his teacher to catch up on his classwork. He was to tell her if he was bullied. His attendance improved, and by the end of the school year, Doug managed to pass fourth grade.

I thoroughly enjoyed Doug's imaginative play and engagement in treatment. He learned that, when a long span of time separated our encounters, he could trigger an appointment by asking his mother when he would see the toy doctor again. He liked the support I offered him. He also managed the timing of the appointments. He liked having his sessions set up at the end of the school day so he would be able to get out early. I wrote a medical excuse so he wasn't marked as absent. After our sessions, he had special one-on-one time with his mother where she would buy him his favorite meal at McDonald's. They would also bring home take-out meals for his brothers.

Our sessions were not regular or consistent during his elementary school years. I would schedule the next session at the end of each appointment, but often Joan would cancel it. Then she would call and schedule another one.

Near the end of Doug's fifth-grade school year, I received a frantic message from his mother. I hadn't seen him for several months. This time she sounded upset on the phone. "Doug wants to come in!" she said. I set up an appointment.

I noticed his sad demeanor and deflated look in the waiting room. He barely made eye contact with me. His pants were unusually worn and ripped, and his hair was disheveled. Black circles ringed his eyes from an obvious lack of sleep.

I encouraged him to come into my office. Instead of going over to the play area, as he normally would, he shuffled over to the chair where his mother usually sat. Clearly, something was bothering him. I asked him what was the matter.

He gathered the courage to share his concerns. "I have never been in that place. It feels like I have to start school all over. I don't want to go. Do I have to?"

I inferred the transition to the larger middle school building for sixth grad-ers was clearly impacting him. He was worried about the change. I knew the anticipation of this change increased his anxiety and impaired his sleep.

I asked him if I could contact his teacher to enlist her help. He happened to like her. Doug responded, "Do you think she could help?" I said I could try to set up a plan to have her on speakerphone during our next session. Maybe she could give us some ideas. He and his mother consented.

* * *

Joan brought him to our next meeting. Doug was perky when he came into my office, as I am sure he wanted help with school. He knew we were going to talk to his teacher. He had become interested in sharks and asked if I could look them up. This was something we often did together, as he always wanted to learn about different animals. I pulled up a site on the internet, and we talked and read about the different kinds of sharks there were in the world. I then had Joan come in, and I asked if Doug was ready for me to call his teacher. I wanted to make sure he was comfortable. He said he was, and I put the phone on the speaker setting and made the call.

With Ms. Tucker on the line, I started the conversation. "Since Doug is here, I thought we could start with some school-related questions. Such as, how does Doug do with his classwork? Does he understand the material? Have you noticed any problems with his peers?"

Ms. Tucker said, "He's a smart boy, and even though he has many absences, he seems to be able to make up his work and catch up with the class. He stays in for recess to finish work if he has to. I know he could do even better if he didn't miss so many school days."

"Do you know if he is being picked on by other students?" I asked. I didn't think he was, as Doug told me he wasn't.

She replied, "I haven't noticed any serious conflicts with his peers. He is a quiet boy and usually stays by himself."

I had previously informed Ms. Tucker about Doug's worries, and now I asked her, "Do you have any ideas to help Doug feel more comfortable about going into the sixth grade?"

She said, "Yes, his guidance counselor and I have come up with a plan."

She described the plan. Over the summer, Doug and his mother would visit the new school on several occasions. During the visits, mother and son would establish relationships with his guidance counselor and teachers. Doug's guidance counselor and teachers would be available to the two of them for questions. He would be able to go into his new classrooms and see what they were like. A tour of the building would happen as well. All attempts would be made to help Doug feel comfortable with the setting.

We thanked Ms. Tucker for her support and her help with the transition. Doug and Joan both appeared to be pleased.

* * *

Doug managed to integrate positively into the sixth grade. However, his middle school years offered new challenges as he struggled to find his identity. He excelled in science, and Mr. Neal, his science teacher, became his mentor. Doug had a knack for understanding animals. He stayed after school and worked with Mr. Neal. He told me Mr. Neal said he should go to college.

He complained in our sessions about other kids bothering him. He shared with me that he felt different from his peers. I encouraged him not to wear the same clothes every day. I suggested that he should use deodorant. He had his mother get him what he needed.

I asked about his friends. He said, "I sit with Sabrina at lunch. She's my only friend. She lives two apartments over from me."

His comparison of students who annoyed him to animals was interesting. He explained it to me this way: "There are certain weaker animals in the herd that don't work together with the herd but pick at the other animals. These are the bullies."

He liked learning different strategies to deal with those peers who annoyed him. Doug was a tall, sturdy boy, and I was concerned he could cause harm to another boy if a conflict escalated. So I had him work on ignoring his peers' nasty comments and letting their words go. He practiced taking a deep, quiet breath while pretending not to hear the bullying words. He later reported his success by telling me, "I learned words don't hurt."

Doug did well academically with the help of Mr. Neal. He told me, "I'm going to be the first one in my family to finish high school." By this time in his treatment, he had developed a work ethic and a sense of commitment. He did have worries about transitioning into high school, though.

"I've never been in the high school building," he said. "It must be like starting a new job. New place, new people, everything is different. Mr. Neal said I have to do well in high school to go to college. Do I really want to go to college?"

Before the start of high school, he asked to come in for a session. The appointment had to be scheduled for later in the day. Joan said to me on the phone, "He told me to set it up after three o'clock. He said that's when he is awake."

Doug usually had a purpose for wanting to come in. This time he wanted to talk about his recent bonding with his father. I didn't fully grasp the meaning of that bond until several years later. This is what he told me at the time.

He said, "I have been spending most of my summer at Dad's. He showed me how he logs. I learned that he has a sixth sense about how to cut trees so it doesn't affect the land. We walked around his many acres. The land was rocky. He has helped me appreciate the outdoors."

"What do you do at your mom's?" I asked.

Doug said, "I play video games there." He was excited to share with me a new game he had traded for. "The game's action takes place in historical settings. It has nice visuals. I like the main character. He's an assassin who fights for peace against figures who want control."

I asked, "Are you ready for school?"

"You know," he said, "I keep thinking about this thing with school, work, and college. I'm not sure about how it comes together for me."

I told him to tell his mother to call me when he was ready to come in again. I wished him well with his new "school job." He laughed and said, "I will see you after school starts."

* * *

I didn't hear from him until the following year. Julie Albright, a state social worker, contacted me. I had worked with her before on other cases. She explained that Doug had been placed in a foster home. Julie said, "Doug was placed in the state's custody due to his excessive school absences. He requested to see you. He said he had seen you in the past for therapy. He told me you were the only one he would talk to."

I told her I would be happy to see Doug again. "What is the case plan?" I asked.

Julie told me the family was assigned a family advocate for support. I consulted weekly to the Family Advocacy Program and knew Wendy, the home-based family worker who would come over to Joan's apartment. She would set up a reunification plan so Doug could return home. The goals to be worked on included the following: regular and consistent school attendance, completing necessary homework, passing his classes, and following curfew and household rules.

I gave Julie an appointment for Doug.

* * *

Joan and Julie brought Doug in for his appointment. Joan was dressed as usual, but Doug had on a new outfit. He immediately stood up when I came into the waiting room and came with me into my office. He was up-front and honest. He said, "I just want to be home. I don't like living in someone else's home." On the positive side, he said, "Sabrina is my girlfriend. I hope they let me see her."

Because of the state's involvement, Doug came to his appointments on a regular basis. He maintained his focus on the reunification objectives so he could return home. He managed to catch up on all his missed work by staying after school. Eventually he went home.

In my weekly consultations with the Family Advocate program, Wendy told me she was assisting Doug with goals to help him become more independent. This was the state's recommendation. She helped him obtain his driver's license. He shared with her his dislike of school, and Wendy, Julie, and Doug met with his guidance counselor. He was placed in a hands-on agricultural and forestry program at the high school. He told me he liked the program. He said he wanted to figure out a way to earn money and not go to college.

"I can raise a pig at Dad's, sell it, and make money," he told me. This was his idea for working. He said, "I think finishing high school is enough for me."

I saw him sporadically. Wendy assisted him in getting a part-time job at a local farm. He worked well with the farmer, and he was given a baby pig. He and his father fed and raised the pig, and when it was grown, his father butchered the animal. Doug traded and sold the parts of the butchered pig.

Wendy closed Doug's case. He did well in his new school program and spent most of his time at his father's home. I lost touch with him for a while, and then his mother called and asked for an appointment for herself and Doug. She said, "I want to know if you can help me get him on disability."

I let her know that now that he was over the age of eighteen, he would have to make the appointment himself. At a later time, he contacted me.

He was quite talkative on the phone. He filled me in about what he had been doing since I last saw him. "I live at Dad's. I raise pigs. I made a farm at his place. I'm so busy all the time, but I really like it. I finished school. I know Mom wants me to sign up for disability. She thinks I need the money. She said we should talk to you about it. I told her I don't need it. I said I would make an appointment anyway. Maybe Dad will come, too. I would like him to meet you."

I set up a scheduled time with him.

The following week, Doug and his parents were sitting together in the waiting room. Doug immediately stood up when I came out. His engaging expression reminded me of the fun times we had when we played together with his favorite animals.

He introduced his father. Slightly shorter than Doug, Big Jeff sported a long, full beard that overshadowed any facial features except for his piercing blue eyes. I'd never expected to meet his father, and I was happy that I finally did.

Doug took charge and guided his parents into my office. Once we were settled, he led the conversation by saying, "I live with him now." He looked at his father, whose eyes widened in agreement.

Looking at Doug, his mother added, "He's having a pig roast. He turned Big Jeff's land into a farm. Wayne helps him. Little Jeff might even come to the roast."

Doug clarified his work and living conditions. "Sabrina and I live with Dad. I sleep better. I get up with the animals. I work the land. We have pigs and chickens. The garden has lettuce, corn, tomatoes, and other vegetables. Sabrina runs the farm stand on the road. Dad butchers the animals. We trade and sell the items. Our pork jerkies are known to be the best."

I had always admired Doug's understanding of animals but wondered how he was able to turn his father's land into a farm. He had said to me before that the area was rocky and would be difficult to farm. I asked him about it.

He said, "The pigs. They clear the land. We block them in an area with logs, and they dig up the rocks looking for food with their noses, much better than a shovel and pick. I move them around, and we now have nice farm land."

I recalled that he said he wanted to earn money by raising pigs. I asked him how he'd been able to do this.

He laughed, "The pigs! The taste of their meat is based on what they eat. I feed them mushrooms. The old apple orchard on our land is loaded with them. I gave the Big Chef—you know, he owns the Chef's Restaurant on the mountain—I gave him some cuts for free to try. He told me the meat is the best he's ever tasted. Now he buys pork chops and ham from me every week."

Doug smiled at me and pulled out a large wad of bills, which he grasped with his left hand and held up with his bent fingers. He said, "Between the logging, the pigs, and the farm, we earn good money."

This prodded his father to make his only statement. He uttered his words softly without hardly moving his mouth. He lifted his head up, and as everyone looked at him, we could see the twinkle in his eyes as he said, "He's sharp like my butcher knife."

The man's bittersweet odor defined him. He had a hearty smell of the woods combined with old sweat from poor hygiene. But his respect for his son was evident—the man Joan said would never talk to a counselor had come to the session.

Joan looked at Doug and asked, "Are you smoking the weed and drinking the moonshine?"

"I don't need any of that," Doug said. "I like what I'm doing. I like the animals, the farm, and working the land."

Joan then turned to me. "Shouldn't he get on disability? Like his older brothers?"

I explained that Doug didn't have severe enough problems to qualify for disability. He had found his own way to work and earn money. "He seems happy with what he has," I said.

"Yeah, he does," his mother agreed. "Doug can take care of himself."

As the session neared its end, Doug asked, "Would you like to come to the pig roast? We're butchering Sausage, and she's one big lady."

At this statement his parents laughed. I then opened the door for them.

The last to leave, Doug grabbed a neatly and colorfully wrapped bag from his jacket pocket and handed it to me. "Here's our best farm-raised pork jerky."

"Who made such a nice package?" I asked.

"Sabrina did."

"I can't wait to try it," I said.

"You're going to enjoy the taste so much you'll want more. Come out to our farm stand and see us. We always have more," Doug replied.

CHALLENGES AND REFLECTIONS

Doug's play was organized, thoughtful, and imaginative. I enjoyed his expressive behavior and his conversation. I was surprised at how much he engaged in our therapy. I didn't expect this after gathering the history from his mother. It was a challenge to explain to her Doug's strengths and potential.

In middle school, his teachers recognized his intelligence. Some encouraged him to pursue college. Doug wanted to satisfy one learning goal—to be the first in his family to graduate high school.

Doug in adolescence put together his imaginative play themes. He liked animals. He wanted to earn money from his interests. He was in high school. He had a family advocacy worker assigned to him because he had missed so many school days. His worker helped him get his first pig. Doug devised a work plan to raise pigs and farm on his father's land.

Doug's father had an alcohol problem. His mother knew it. Doug understood the problem. In therapy, Doug admitted he didn't want to repeat his father's drinking behavior. Doug instead bonded with his father on their mutual connection to nature and the land.

Chapter 10

Mandy's Psychological Dilemmas

PRESENTING PROBLEMS

Mandy was moving out of her family's household at the end of the summer. She was going to graduate school to study psychology. She wanted a therapy experience. This would be her first time in therapy. She was twenty-one years old. She didn't present with any specific treatment goals.

Mandy's research plan was to study the effects of family patterns on behavior. I talked with her about the importance of having therapy goals. She became interested in exploring her own psychological family patterns. We scheduled a short-term therapy intervention for the summer.

In treatment she talked about her mother's and father's character strengths and weaknesses. She realized they were part of her psychology, too. She became aware that she learned to act in a similar fashion to them. She believed that her parents' patterns of interactions were intertwined with hers. This made her worry about her choices in intimate relationships.

In our brief therapeutic time, she evaluated her career plans. She realized something about leaving her home and family. She came to the conclusion that she wouldn't be able to forget her family. Their behavior patterns would continue to have an effect on her.

TREATMENT STORY

When I first met Mandy in the waiting room, she was dressed in a pant-suit, and her warm facial expression was engaging. This was not what I had expected after our conversation on the phone last week, when I got the impression that she would be more serious and formal.

"My name is Mandy," she had said to me on the phone. "I have completed my senior year at college with high honors. I am starting a PhD in clinical psychology in the fall. I want to schedule eight sessions of therapy over the summer before I leave for California to attend graduate school. I am only available on Monday or Tuesday evenings."

I asked her during our call if she had ever been in therapy before. She told me she hadn't been, but she wanted to see what it was like. She said she has been pursuing a research degree but hadn't ruled out being a therapist.

I introduced myself to her in the waiting room. I explained the paperwork to her. She was attentive to the material and asked several questions about the forms. After she completed the information, I showed her into my office.

I usually didn't have patients coming into therapy for a learning experience. I wondered if she might have some issues she wanted to address. We all have to face our psychological dilemmas. I began the session with these thoughts in mind.

* * *

Once we were settled in the office, Mandy said, "You came highly recommended by my primary care physician. I think my reason for seeking therapy at this time has something to do with my family and my career plans."

I was curious if she had some parent, sibling, or other relationship conflict. I asked, "Are you comfortable telling me about your family?"

"I have Japanese and American heritage," she said. "My mother met my father when he was stationed in Okinawa. They relocated to the United States after they were married. I feel more a part of the American culture, but my mother still doesn't want to integrate into this society." She continued, "We moved to this area when I was an infant. I was born in Japan. My little sister was born here. My father is employed as an engineer for a local company."

I became intrigued by her cultural differences. I was curious how she dealt with her parents' contrasting cultural values. Her face showed a combination of Japanese and American characteristics. I asked, "How does your mother handle the culture here?"

She replied, "She wanted to teach calligraphy in Japan, but since moving to America she's been like a stay-at-home mother. She maintains contact with some friends here of Japanese heritage. She does her art at home in her studio. Her work is unique."

"What makes her art so unusual?" I could see Mandy was appreciative of her mother's work.

"She combines calligraphy styles and color to show emotions and feelings through her designs. I like looking at her pieces," Mandy said.

"What about your father?" I asked. She described her mother as an artist, and admiration and affection were apparent. I was interested in how she would describe her father.

"My father is devoted to his career and works long hours. He's a successful engineer. He spends a lot of time at the company headquarters in San Francisco. He's rarely at home," she said.

I reminded her that she stated over the phone that she would like to be in therapy for a brief period over the summer. She would be moving to California to start graduate school after that. I still didn't feel I had an understanding of why she was seeking help. I needed more information. I asked her, "Do you have any specific treatment goals?"

"I was thinking that maybe I could gain a better understanding of my family relationships and family patterns. I believe that therapy might help me with this."

"How does that tie into your career?" I wondered.

"I decided to come in for therapy at this time since I haven't ruled out becoming a therapist," Mandy said. "I wanted to see what it was like. I haven't chosen whether to continue to do research or enter a clinical internship at the end of my program and do therapy. I have a research topic, which is to study learned family patterns."

I was struck by her insight. "You have an idea that would tie your research into your own personal experience," I said. I thought her research topic was compelling. What about her family patterns? Which of her relationships would she be ready to talk about first? Her mother's, her father's, or her sister's? I asked, "How do you see your family relationships?"

"Yes," she said, "you're right. I need to look at my own family. I think I would like to talk about my mother as our relationship is the least complicated."

"That's an interesting way of describing your interactions with your mother," I said. But it left me even more curious about her relationship with her father.

Smiling, she opened up about her mother. "My mother has always been warm and caring and devoted to my father. She continues to create Japanese art using her knowledge of calligraphy, but not for money. My father had a studio built for her. She spends many hours in the studio painting. Our major conflict is that I believe it's important for women to have a career to earn their own money and not just be financially dependent on their husbands. After many debates, my mother has been supportive of my decision to have a career—it's the American way of life, she would say."

"So it appears you and your mother have come to some sort of understanding," I observed.

"I would agree with that," she said. "I can talk honestly to my mother, even though we have divergent values about women and work. We can accept each other's differences."

"What about your younger sister? What sort of relationship do you have with her?" I figured talking about her sister might be less intrusive in this first session than addressing her relationship with her father.

Mandy shut her eyes as if conjuring an image of her sister in her mind. She said, "Jane and I get along, but it's almost as if we have opposite purposes. She wants to be an artist and enjoy life. We have fun together, but she says I'm too uptight and I need to loosen up."

I wondered if her sister might have a point—Mandy seemed very driven. Was she able to have some fun? "What do you think about what your sister said?" I asked.

She said, "I think she may be right somewhat. I worked hard in college and have graduated with special honors, and I am faithful to my studies. My sister likes to go out and socialize. She thinks work should be fun. She doesn't approve of my intense work ethic."

"Do you feel your sister may have some perspective on your behavior?" I asked, hoping Mandy would at least take into account what her sister was saying. As we talked about her family, she sat straight up, not touching the back of her chair, with her feet squarely planted on the rug. She appeared to have trouble relaxing.

"Well, sure, I'm devoted to my studies." She said, "This is one of the conflicts in my family. My sister and my mother bond, mostly around art. Supposedly, I'm more like my father. My father is consumed by his work. I have considered what Jane says about me. Since starting college, I've made an effort to become involved socially and have fun. I even dated, and I have had a couple of relationships. Nothing special, though; I'm not ready for that."

I noted that our time was almost up, and I reviewed what we had discussed. I said we could look more at her family later. Since she was thinking about being a therapist and this was her first therapy session, I asked her, "What do you think about being in therapy?"

She moved back into the chair and clasped her hands. "I feel like I have been given the chance to reflect on myself and explain who I am." She said, "The therapy process feels very overwhelming and powerful. Things that I have thought and worried about seem to take on a new meaning when I say them. It seems to me that when I clearly describe and express my feelings into words, the words take on a different meaning from the thoughts I have had about myself."

I thanked her for sharing about her therapy experience. Her personal statements left an interesting conclusion to end our first time together. I scheduled an appointment with her for the following week.

* * *

At our next session, Mandy was initially standoffish and seemed resistant to talking about herself. I think she felt she revealed too much during our last visit. I decided to lighten up the conversation and asked, "How was your weekend?"

She said, "Now that my college studies are finished, I've been working full time this summer to save money. I waitressed this past weekend. I'm always willing to do extra shifts so I can have spending money for graduate school. Whatever free time I have I spend with Anna and Carrie. They've been my girlfriends for a long time. I worked at Carrie's mother's day care for my first part-time job in high school."

I thought this would be a way to understand her social connections. I knew that people who grew up in a rural area tended to maintain a small group of friends throughout their school years. I figured exploring her friendships would be helpful. I asked, "Are you going to miss your friends when you leave?"

She said, "The three of us started getting close in seventh grade. We went to the same schools. I think I'll miss them. We even went to the same local college."

I was interested in learning about her social life. I wanted to get at the type of interactions she had with her friends. I knew if she could talk about the kind of relationships she had with them it might help identify more about her character. "How would you describe your friendships?"

She considered my question before responding. "I think I'm the helper," she said. "My girlfriends would confide in me. They trusted me because I could keep secrets. I made a commitment to not talk about them behind their backs. I would offer them help and advice. Which was why I thought about being a therapist!"

I wondered how she handled this role with her friends. A lot of teenage bonding focuses on criticizing others in order to bond against a targeted individual. How did she balance trust and loyalty in her friendships? I realized the helper role could be difficult to maintain consistently. What made her commit to this position? I believed her friendship narrative was important to pursue. "What was it like being in a helping role?"

She stayed collapsed in her chair, and after deliberating, she said, "I like helping others. I feel that when I assist others, it helps me feel good about myself. I think I have been placed in problematic binds in the past by keeping shared information private."

I had touched on something. She must have a memory of such a difficult situation. Would she be able to disclose the conflict? She was beginning to be honest about her relationships, so I asked, "Do you remember a situation where keeping secrets wasn't helpful?"

"I remember several years ago when Anna was dating this guy Josh in college. We would all hang out together with him and his friends. They lived in the dorms while Anna, Carrie, and I were all commuters. We would sometimes stay at the dorms for the weekend. I even became involved with one of his friends. Carrie confided in me that she really liked Josh and didn't know what to do. She wanted to know what I thought. We talked a lot about her feelings for him. She eventually confided in me she was sleeping with Josh, too. I didn't know what to do."

"So you were caught in a bind with your friends," I said. "How did you handle the situation?" I wanted to attempt to gain some perspective on how she solved problems in her relationships. How did she manage her social commitments?

She said, "I had made a pact with myself to be honest with my friends. But I was also a strong believer in not sharing a friend's story with another friend when it was told to me in confidence. I was conflicted. I told Carrie she needed to tell Josh that he had to tell Anna about their relationship."

"How did it work out?" I asked. "You're still friends with both of them."

"It has entangled mine and Anna's friendship to this day."

"How so?"

"I believe the divide in our friendships happened because Carrie decided to tell Anna what was going on after several months. Josh apparently refused to be truthful and continued sleeping with the both of them. Anna found out I had known about the whole thing since it began and was extremely hurt that I never told her. She said to me, *What kind of friendship do we have?* I still remember her words when she said she'd never be able to completely trust me again. I felt so sad that I had lost a close friend."

"What a conflict," I said. "Why did you keep Carrie's story a secret for so long?" I had begun to be curious about this dynamic and whether there was more to it.

She admitted, "I struggled with wanting to tell Anna, but I believed it wasn't my right. The longer it went on, the more tense our relationship became. I could feel a lack of closeness. I thought, *why was I keeping such a secret from her?* I recall I couldn't take it anymore. I pressured Carrie to tell her. But it was too late. The wedge remains in the place between Anna and me, even today. Our friendship will never be the same. I'm ready to move on and leave for graduate school and meet new friends."

"What kinds of friendships are you looking for?"

"I think my friendships should be for having fun and doing fun things together. But honesty and trust are important to me, too. But if I'm going to be a helper, I'll do it as a therapist."

We had talked about friendships and loyalty. Next, Mandy asked me about the therapeutic relationship. She wanted to know more about how I maintained trust and honesty as a therapist. I explained that the basis of this was the ethical commitment to confidentiality and privacy. I presented her with the following example. "Because you and I are living in a small community,

I could easily run into you at the farmers market. Since I am known as a therapist, I wouldn't acknowledge you unless you said something to me first. It would therefore be up to you to disclose the relationship. I wouldn't recognize you without your social consent. If we spoke, it would only be in generalities and not about anything personal."

"Do social relationships have guidelines?" she thought out loud. "For instance, if I ran into a friend at the farmers market, we would talk with each other."

I said that she was correct. However, I continued, whether she engages more in the conversation or just leaves to do her shopping was her choice. Whereas we had preestablished rules in a therapeutic relationship, she had to establish her own rules in social interactions. If she wanted to have a more intimate relationship, she would have to pursue a more in-depth and trusting interaction.

"You're right," Mandy said, "The decisions I make about relationships are based on my beliefs. If I want honest friendships, it's up to me. But long-term partners have to be able to trust each other."

I told her that, even after she moved away and established new relationships, she would have to decide on the quality of the friendships she wanted to have.

"I have a lot to think about with my moving away," Mandy said. "I feel better that we talked about my friendships."

* * *

Several sessions later Mandy came in wearing a long, colorful red dress. She told me it was a kimono that her mother recently bought for her. She seemed angry even though the outfit made her look elegant. Mandy said, "I feel bothered because my father just left for his regular business trip to California. He goes for close to a month. It always upsets me when he goes. He's done this since I can remember, but it still gives me a bad feeling."

Was there something behind her worries? I asked, "Do you recall some old anxieties about your father leaving?"

Mandy thought about this and offered a memory. "My father has always gone away for long periods of time. I worry, though. I think it relates to a confrontation I had with him when I was in high school. I might have been fifteen. It was when he had returned from one of his trips. He and my mother had an argument. I overheard it. It sounded like my mother was sobbing. This was unusual. They never had fights."

As she continued talking, there was tension in her face, and her body turned rigid. This was the appearance I had noticed at our first meeting. It had since subsided, as she had become more relaxed talking about her family.

"The next day after my parents' fight, I knocked on my mother's drawing studio door. She said I could come in. Oftentimes when I would ask to come in, she would be pleasant and would show me her work. This time I remember being transfixed by the piece she was sketching. The lines were droopy, and the quality of the blue hues had such a sad and depressing feeling. Her drawings usually had an upbeat feeling with strong designs and bright colors. This piece was strikingly different. She was crying. I asked her what was the matter. She said she didn't like it when my father went away. She felt lonely. She told me he sees another woman when he goes. She said she asked him if he would ever leave her. He told her he was committed to their marriage and that was all she needed to know. The look on her face and the image of her drawing left an impression on me to this day. I understood her despair and felt so much a part of it."

She sat back in the chair and took a deep inhale and exhale before going on. "I sat with my mother's statements for a while. I decided I didn't like what my father had told her. It felt like he was not being totally honest with her. I thought I should approach him about the argument, too. Since I asked my mother about the fight, why not ask my father what happened? I think I was expecting him to be sincere when I talked with him. So I went to him. I said I heard them arguing and I heard my mother crying. And I directly asked him if he was involved with another woman. He never clearly responded—he avoided the question. He told me he and my mother had a good marriage and I should stay out of it. His words were that their marriage was *not my concern*." She made air quotes with her fingers at these last words. She added, "After that, I realized we would never be able to have a totally honest relationship."

She thought some and continued, "This experience with my parents helped me understand their relationship. They had a commitment to each other as part of the marriage. But the concept of an honest, exclusive, and trusting relationship wasn't part of their marriage. Because my father wouldn't be clear with me or my mother about having an affair, I felt I couldn't trust him. I decided I wasn't going to be like that. The idea of keeping secrets—that was not going to happen for me."

I wondered more about her father. I asked, "Is there a pattern of infidelity in your family?"

"My father's father divorced my grandmother after my parents married. My mother says my grandfather cheated on my grandmother; she died about a year later. My mother refuses to see him to this day. My father visits him when he travels."

I asked, "What is your relationship like with your father?"

"He's supporting my career, and he has helped me with finances. He reviewed my applications, made comments, and went with me on college visits. He even researched the various fields of psychology, developed spreadsheets with pros and cons about the profession, and has been an instrumental part of my decisions. We actually get along very well as long as we don't discuss anything personal. Mother has taken a back seat and has not been involved in my future plans. So maybe that's why I said my father and I have a complex relationship. We can discuss certain things in detail but have significant limitations in our other interactions. He never asks about my friends, and I can't talk about Mother with him. And I can never talk to him about his other relationship."

"The fact that you feel your parents don't have a deep, exclusive commitment to each other affects the trust you have in long-term relationships," I said.

Mandy appeared startled and said, "Yes! Secrets! That's what caused the conflict between Anna and Carrie! I wasn't being fully honest! Instead, by keeping secrets, I did the same thing my parents have done with each other. My father keeps his other relationship a secret. This is going to be hard work learning to not repeat destructive family patterns."

I said, "Reflecting on your actions is sometimes difficult but can also be revealing." The session ended after this.

* * *

After I returned from my two-week summer vacation, we had another scheduled appointment. I noticed when Mandy came into my office that she looked like she was bothered or upset. At first I was concerned that it might be because of the lapse in our treatment. I asked, "Are you okay?"

"I've been feeling angry that my father has left again. But I'm more worried that I will be leaving soon. I was thinking it was the last summer home before I move away."

I asked, "What do you, your sister, and mother usually do when your father is away?" These trips had happened since she was a child. What was it like for her and her family without her father?

"I remember when I was a child and he left. My mother seemed different. She would do fun stuff with us. She would have us do art projects in her studio. She would make special Japanese meals for us. This past week my mother was great. She prepared my favorite dish. The three of us have been enjoying our time together. It makes me not want to leave."

Mandy described in detail the dish her mother made for her. "It's her special miso soup. She serves it in a bowl of wheat noodles with green onions, seaweed, and pieces of pork."

"I wouldn't mind tasting that," I said. "I can see how your father dominates the family. Your mother seems like a creative, playful person. Are you going to miss her?"

"Yes, very much so! Her warmth and care has helped me a lot. But I have to move on. I want something different in my life. I can't stay. I feel if I don't move away, I won't grow up. I need to discover new things. If I remain here it will stifle me. Mother and I will find our way to stay close."

"Leaving your family is hard. Do you have any regrets?" I wondered.

"I feel disappointed in my parents' marriage. It's not what I want. I think I have to continue working on being honest in my friendships. Boys try too much to control you! I think I have to find a more equal relationship. I don't see that with my parents. My father has too much control!"

"I see you have made a commitment to not repeat some of the negative patterns in your family," I said.

"Maybe that's another reason I have to move away," she said. "I need the change! A new perspective, I guess. I feel I have learned to be confident by being open and direct. When I'm around my parents, I can't be up front. I can be more honest with Mother, but I feel limitations in what can be said. I realize no family is perfect, and I see the imperfections in my family."

"At least you're excited about your studies," I said. "You will be moving away to develop your career."

Mandy spoke more about her interest in studying psychology. She explained, "Deciding whether to go into research or become a therapist is one of my many dilemmas. But I have several years before I have to make that commitment."

I said, "You have choices to make about your career and family patterns you might want to change."

"I have to work on not repeating my parents' negative patterns. I'm ready to move on with my own life. Time to grow up. It's up to me to find my way."

I asked, "What do you have left to do before you move?" I wondered if her father would come home to help.

"Mother and Jane are helping me," she said. "We have a shopping trip planned for this weekend. I'll ship my stuff. My father plans to meet me when I'm on campus."

We closed our session and scheduled a final meeting before she would leave the area for graduate studies.

* * *

At our last session, Mandy had finished most of her preparations to move. She was wearing a new shirt with the name of her graduate school on it. She was leaving her job and was planning a special weekend getaway with Carrie and Anna. They were going to Anna's family cabin in the mountains. It was a significant transition time for her, so I asked if she would like for us to summarize her brief treatment experience.

I started. "If I recall correctly, you told me that you wanted some help understanding the impact your family relationships have had on you." I asked, "Do you think you have accomplished this goal?"

Mandy said, "I think I realize relationships mean commitments, which means I have to work at them. I know trust will always be an issue for me. I think it's because of the mistrust I have experienced."

I said I could see how her father's affair continued to trouble her.

I asked whether spending a short time in therapy herself had helped her decide about becoming a therapist.

She replied, "I've already submitted a research proposal as part of my application. I have some time to decide on becoming a therapist. I plan to investigate how patterns such as poverty, violence, mental illness, trauma, and divorce are repeated in family systems. I want to demonstrate how psychological concerns are a complex of patterns and learned behaviors that repeat in families over generations." She smiled and continued, "I think my own therapy experience has been helpful. It makes me think more about being a therapist."

I said her research topic should provide her with insights into working with family patterns. I reminded her that she will have several years in the PhD program before she will have to decide about starting her clinical training to be a therapist.

She added, "I like the idea of family patterns of behavior. I believe there must be both negative and positive learned interactions. As a therapist, maybe I could help people sort out the family system. Then, I could help them so they don't repeat the negative actions."

"You have been able to discover patterns in your own family," I said.

Mandy said, "Yes! Being a therapist would allow me to combine my father's scientific qualities as well as my mother's artistic side. My mother worked with me on a piece of art that I want to hang in my new space. I believe there is an artistic rhythm in the therapeutic relationship. I think people have patterns in their relationships. Like the design patterns I see in my mother's art."

I said I could see that she was thinking more about what it would be like being a therapist. I said it also seemed that she was beginning to look into some of her family's positive aspects as well as her family's problems. I noted that moving away from her family meant more growing up and learning to find herself.

"I have to be careful not to forget about my upbringing. It will always be a part of me. This means I can continue to learn from my childhood by understanding the good and not-so-good patterns I have experienced."

"Learning about yourself will be helpful in being a good therapist," I commented.

Mandy said, "I have been reading a lot about being a therapist. I'm learning from my studies. The more I'm in touch with myself, the better helper I'll be."

I wondered aloud, "Have you thought about the age-group and population you might possibly be interested in working with when you graduate?"

She said, "I was thinking about children. When I worked in Carrie's mother's day care for a short time, I really liked playing with the children."

"I really like doing play therapy with children," I said. "I believe it can give you the same meditative experience that you describe your mother enjoying with her art."

"Maybe being a child therapist could help me balance my interests."

"In the future, I plan to write a book about what it is like being a child psychologist," I said. "I would like to include your story."

"How would my story fit in?" she asked.

I said that she had done a terrific job of recognizing her psychological dilemmas at this time in her life. I explained that this will help her in the future make the kinds of choices and decisions she needs to undertake after she leaves her family and lives on her own. I said I would like to use her story to show how even after one grows out of childhood and adolescence, the patterns of their childhood still create dilemmas for them to work on later in life.

"My dilemmas, my choices, understanding my family's patterns and making decisions about my career and my relationships based on that knowledge," she said. "I think I see."

I explained that I would make every effort to protect her privacy and confidentiality. I told her that I hoped my book would encourage more people to become child therapists. We finished our session with this review of her treatment experience.

CHALLENGES AND REFLECTIONS

An important challenge of psychotherapy is to establish a goal for treatment. Mandy came into therapy without a clear plan. She had never been in therapy before. She wanted to see what it was like. Mandy was thinking about becoming a therapist. But she hadn't reflected on her own life.

Our brief therapeutic relationship was based on helping Mandy understand the dynamics of her family. She became invested in learning about how her parents' actions had an effect on her behavior. This was what she wanted to study in graduate school. She examined her parents' positive and negative behavior patterns. This was her mission in our treatment.

Mandy saw similarities in her own behaviors to her parents. She realized the rigorous devotion to her academic study was something she had gotten from her father. Her playful side and the joy she had found working with children was from her mother. She worried about her parents' negative patterns. She recalled that her parents didn't have a secure, exclusive, and trusting marriage. This shattered her belief in the sacredness of their relationship. It had made her think about whether she would be able to trust a close relationship.

Mandy hoped that by leaving home she would be able to find herself. She wanted to become a mature and responsible adult. She wanted to begin her own life and establish her career. Mandy had plans to study the generational effects of patterns such as violence, divorce, and substance abuse have on families while in graduate school. Little had she realized that her parents' positive and negative behaviors could have a significant impact on her own behavior and thinking. She realized that even the subtle factor of her parents' unhealthy marriage might have an effect on her ability to trust relationships.

Discussion Questions

CHAPTER 1: DOES RICKY HAVE DEPRESSION?

1. Why were Ricky's attention problems seen initially as depression or as acting out behaviors?
2. Why did Autumn and Rick see Ricky's attention issues differently? How did they eventually come to understand his problems? Why was Autumn Ricky's best advocate?
3. Why was the classroom so frustrating for Ricky? What skills did Ricky learn in therapy that helped with his focusing during school?
4. Was the medication intervention helpful? How did the medication help Ricky?
5. How did having a 504 plan help Ricky at school? Why was it important to work with the school?
6. What were some of the significant transitions in Ricky's treatment?
7. How did Ricky begin to take responsibility for his attention problems?
8. Do you think Ricky, as a young adult, still had attention issues? What had he learned from his therapy to help him in his job?

CHAPTER 2: RAINBOW DASH

1. Why did Arlene want James in therapy?
2. What behaviors were observed in James that were consistent with autism spectrum disorder?
3. What were the best ways to connect with James in therapy?
4. What is gender creative play therapy?
5. How did Arlene come to understand James's behavioral differences?
6. What were the early signs of James's gender identity? Why was it important to explore gender differences in therapy?
7. How was social media important for James?

8. How was the process of James's transition to Jamie handled in therapy? Why was it important to use the appropriate pronouns for Jamie?
9. What was the significance of gender-confirming surgery for Jamie?

CHAPTER 3: ANGRY DAN

1. Why was Beth so concerned about Dan's anger?
2. What effect did Larry's actions have on Dan?
3. How did Dan exhibit his angry behaviors in play therapy?
4. How did Dan understand his actions through the play therapy interventions?
5. What did Beth learn about parenting Dan?
6. What complicated Dan's behavior in adolescence when he was dividing his time between Beth's and Larry's households?
7. Why was Larry resistant to treatment?
8. How did the past experience of violence and the use of substances contribute to Dan's arrest?
9. Why was the forensic evaluation helpful in Dan's situation? Why was it important to communicate with the forensic evaluator as a part of the treatment with Dan?

CHAPTER 4: THE TRAUMA BINDER

1. Why did Javon and Jasmine experience their early trauma differently during developmental transitions?
2. How did Javon's early trauma experience affect his play? How was Javon's trauma addressed in play therapy?
3. How did Jasmine's early experience with men affect her relationships as she developed?
4. How did Javon begin to show confidence by dealing with racial prejudice?
5. What did Jasmine mean that she had "awakened from her trauma"?
6. Why was it important to revisit Javon's and Jasmine's early trauma experience as adolescents? How was this dealt with in family therapy?
7. Why was the trauma binder effective in helping Peggy deal with her grandchildren's trauma? How was it helpful to the children?
8. Why did Javon and Jasmine want to detach from their mother?
9. What were the co-therapy strategies in this case?

CHAPTER 5: THE DOLLHOUSE

1. Did the early loss of Jenny's biological parents have later psychological effects?
2. What was the importance of an adoptive family for Jenny?
3. How did "holding therapy" affect Jenny's treatment?
4. Were Tina and Miriam good parents for Jenny? Why?
5. What troubles did Jenny have with her present relationships that brought her into therapy?
6. Why did Jenny's experience of loneliness present an ongoing theme in her development?
7. What did the dollhouse mean to Jenny?
8. How did Jenny learn to accept her adoption in therapy?
9. How was Jenny able to improve her relationships?

CHAPTER 6: THE PROBLEM OF DIVORCE

1. What were the co-therapy strategies used to deal with this divorced family?
2. How did the structure of divorce and having two different households affect Dominic, Bradley, and Mariah? How was each child affected?
3. How did Nicole's and Gary's feelings toward each other contribute to their children's problems?
4. What was the problem with Nicole and Gary's custody agreement and visitation arrangement as the children aged and developed?
5. How did Dominic express his concerns about the divorce in therapy?
6. Why was the family session with Mariah and her mother a transition in the family's treatment?
7. What were the changes Nicole and Gary realized that they needed to make for the benefit of their children?
8. Did Nicole and Gary's engagement in divorce-related family therapy change their relationship? What were the co-therapy approaches used to work with Nicole and Gary's relationship in their therapy sessions together?

CHAPTER 7: ARTY'S SECRET WINNER

1. What important role did Misty have in Arty's childhood?
2. How did Arty deal with Sherry's mental illness?
3. How did Arty's father make matters more difficult for Arty?

4. What caused Arty's resistance to therapy?
5. What behaviors put Arty at risk as an adolescent?
6. Why did Misty lose trust in Arty?
7. Was a residential treatment facility the best alternative for Arty? What was helpful and not helpful for Arty in this self-contained environment?
8. How did Misty and Arty's relationship change during his adolescence? Why did Misty decide to give Arty another chance?

CHAPTER 8: SAM AND SHIRA

1. Why did Emily decide Sam and Shira needed therapy?
2. Why did Emily miss the cues about Nick? How did Shira and Sam deal with Nick's actions?
3. Why did Shira and Sam show different behaviors in school after the incident happened with Nick?
4. What should parents teach their children about sexuality and boundaries?
5. How did Emily's childhood affect her parenting?
6. Why was it important therapeutically and ethically to include Emily in making the child abuse report?
7. What made Emily commit to raising her children differently? Did Emily change her relationships with males?
8. What was the family treatment like after the report was made?

CHAPTER 9: IS DOUG DISABLED?

1. Why wasn't Joan's purpose for wanting Doug in therapy clear?
2. Why was it important to gather a thorough family history from Joan?
3. What was the quality of Doug's play early in treatment?
4. What made a sleep intervention a good first therapeutic goal?
5. What were Doug's issues with school?
6. How was Doug different from the rest of his family?
7. What happened when Doug's family got involved with the state's child abuse and neglect system?
8. How did growing up in poverty affect Doug's development?
9. Could Doug be considered successful in his life and work?

CHAPTER 10: MANDY'S PSYCHOLOGICAL DILEMMAS

1. Why was it important for Mandy to establish some therapy goals at the beginning of treatment?
2. What kind of relationship did Mandy have with her father? How would you describe Mandy's relationship with her mother?
3. How could Mandy's father's infidelity have a psychological effect on her later intimate relationships?
4. What patterns of behavior did Mandy learn from her father and her mother?
5. Was Mandy's research proposal valid? Do families have patterns of behavior that are repeated? What did Mandy learn about her own psychological family patterns of behavior?
6. What kinds of insights did Mandy gain from her short-term therapy experience?
7. Could Mandy be a good therapist?

Index

About the Author

Louis Propp, PsyD, is a clinical psychologist who has been in private practice for almost forty years. He conducts weekly online supervision for home-based workers and maintains a small teletherapy practice in Maine. He has also consulted for almost thirty-five years for a family resource center in Vermont. He has previously taught different graduate-level psychology courses in child psychology at Antioch University New England. He is a member of the Maine, Vermont, and American Psychological Associations, as well as the Association of State and Provincial Psychology Boards.

He completed his doctor of psychology (PsyD) degree at the University of Denver in 1982, where his specialty was clinical child psychology. During his graduate years, he presented various research papers and published his doctoral paper in the *Journal of Child and Adolescent Psychotherapy.*

His first position was in upstate New York, doing play therapy in a school for emotionally disturbed children. In 1984, he became director of a satellite community mental health clinic in Vermont. After three years, he left the clinic and joined a small private practice group. In the 1990s, he helped transition the group into a large, multi-specialty practice to deal with the restrictions of managed care. In 2010, with his wife, Kristin, he formed a private practice focused on children, adolescents, and families. They relocated the practice to the state of Maine in 2020 during the COVID-19 pandemic. Dr. Propp continues to see patients remotely in Vermont and Maine.

9 781538 190371